EXPLAINING HEALTH

What YOU Need to Know
to Stay Healthy

MARCIA M. DEGELMAN
Integrative Medicine Specialist

acknowledgements:

I wish to thank everyone who has helped me on this journey; all of clients over the years, who have shared their wisdom with me. I'd also like to thank my family for their patience and understanding when I had to close the door in order to write this book.

ISBN 978-0-9838497-0-4

BE WELL ✦ PRESS
SAN FRANCISCO

Table of Contents

Part I
Healthy Habits
What is Health...2
Healthcare...3
Lifespan...4
Telomeres...5
Self talk...6
Attitude...7
Three Pillars of Health...8
Ten easy changes...9
Relaxation...10
Healthy Aging...11

Food
Okinawan Foods...15
Mediterranean Foods...16
Essential Fatty Acids...18
Antioxidants...22
Vitamins...24
Benefits of Fiber...28
Fermented Foods...29
Benefits of Soy...30
Benefits of Tea...32
Calcium...34

Exercise
Benefits of Exercise...37
Yoga...42
Tai chi...44
Pilates...46

Sleep
How Much ...50
Insomnia Strategies...52
Progressive Relaxation...53
Self Massage...54
Sleep Hygiene...55
Visualization...56

Part II
Dangers and Defenses
Stress...60
Heart Health...65
Immune system...74
Illnesses...80
Heart Attack,,,80
Cancer...81
Stroke...83
Diabetes...84
Environmental Illness...86

Part III
Other Geographies
Chinese Medicine...88
Ayurveda...98

Part IV
Personal Care
Ergonomics...110
Massage Therapy...112
Bodywork...114
Home Remedies...116
Strains and Sprains...117
When to Use Ice/Heat...118
Colds & Flu...119
Coughs...122

Part V
Mind/Body
Power Down...124
Ways to Be Happy...126
Pleasure and Happiness...128
Mindfulness...131
Guided Visualization132
Meditation133
Recommendations...135
References...136

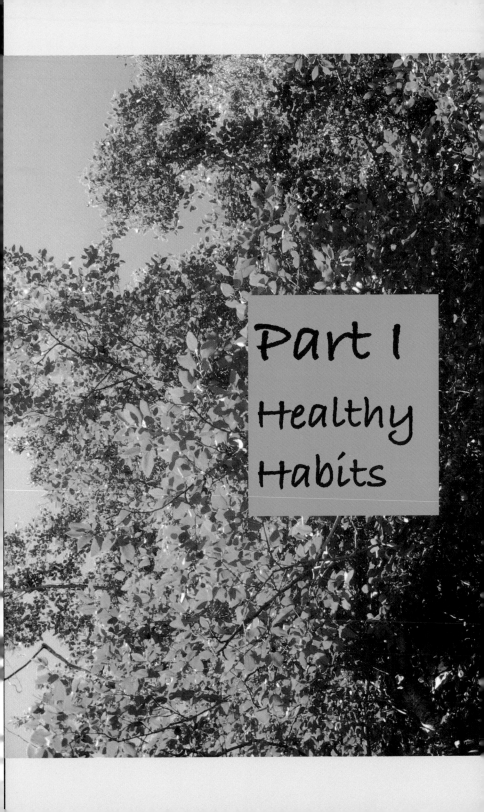

Part I
Healthy Habits

What is health?

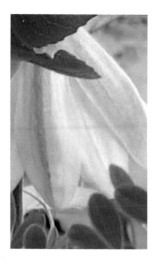

We have to be responsible for our own health

health span
It's not how many years you live—it's how healthy you are the years that you live.

Healthy habits make the difference.

Health is a feeling of vitality, of resilience, not just the absence of disease. Health is having the mental, emotional and physical resources to handle whatever life deals us.

Life hands us some cards at birth. Some come from the environment, our family of origin, and our early health habits. Some get dealt to us along the way, through relationships, good and bad, injuries, illnesses. What's important is not what happens to us; **it's how we handle it.**

How we handle stress is especially important. If we live everyday as if it's an emergency, and get upset over things like traffic, which we have no control over, we will wear ourselves out.

Medicine today can keep us alive longer, but it is up to us to make it a long, healthy life. Choices you make today will influence your health tomorrow.

Healthcare

We have to learn how to become our own health advocates. We have to make our own health care choices. We have to educate ourselves about all of the options and choices available.

We have to become savvy consumers of information found on the internet. There's a lot of information out there, but it's not all reliable. Look at the site and see if it is trying to sell you something. The more reliable sites end in .org, .edu or .gov.

Individuals vary and so do treatments. There are other medical systems besides the western allopathic system. If you have an acute injury or trauma, go to the hospital. For some chronic pain or discomfort, look into alternatives like acupuncture or massage therapy.

There is very little about health in our healthcare system. It's really more of a disease care system.

The medical system has become too specialized, too compartmentalized. There is no one looking out for the whole person, body, mind, and spirit.

We are spending enormous amounts on technology for diagnosing, symptom alleviation and chronic disease management that, for a large part, is created by a sedentary, stress-filled lifestyle.

Lifespan

Everything has a natural life span

Fruit flies live a few days

Mice live about 3 years

Dogs and cats live 15-20 years

Gorillas live 25-35 years

Some trees live for thousands of years

Human lifespan is 80-120 years

Life expectancy

Before 1900 the average life expectancy was 47 years. Most people died of infectious diseases. Thanks to improved public health and modern medicine, the average life expectancy in the U.S. today is 74 years for men and 80 years for women.

Leading causes of death

Heart disease, cancer, stroke, pneumonia, influenza and diabetes are the leading causes of death in the U.S. Some of these are degenerative diseases that can be affected by the way you live—diet, exercise, attitude, and the way you respond to stress.

Centenarians

In 1980 there were 15,000 centenarians (people 100 years old or older) in the U.S. In 2000, there were 77,000. In 2050, there are projected to be 834,000 people living to be 100 years old or more. If you want to be one of them, you need to take care of your health now.

Santrock, John. <u>Life-span Development</u>

4

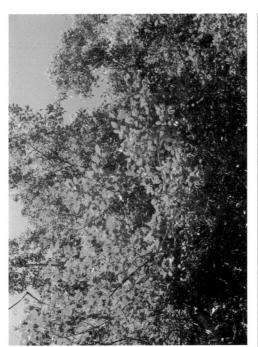

Telomeres
Every cell is programmed to divide a set number of times. The end of a chromosome is a telomere, like the tip of a shoelace. Each time the cell divides the telomere gets shorter. When it gets too short, the cell stops dividing and dies.

Antioxidants
can help cells avoid damage, not divide as often,and live longer.

Inflammation
Many chronic diseases have underlying inflammation. Anti-inflammatory fats, like omega-3 found in fish oil can help reduce inflammation.

Healthy habits practiced daily can help lead to a healthy future

Weil, Andrew, MD. <u>Healthy Aging</u>

5

Self talk

The first step towards health is becoming aware of what we are saying to ourselves. Pay attention to the tone of self talk. Are you putting yourself down, or are you encouraging yourself? Are you taking credit for good things in your life or are you blaming yourself when things go wrong?

Optimism

Optimists have stronger immune systems, and live longer, healthier lives.

Optimists take credit for the good things and expect them to last, while seeing setbacks as temporary, not blaming themselves, not letting it affect their self-esteem.

We can all learn to be optimists by challenging negative thought patterns and replacing them with positive thoughts. We all have inner strength and resilience. We need to find ways to cultivate inner strength in ourselves.

Seligman, Martin <u>Learned Optimism</u>

Attitude

Have an optimistic attitude about life. View difficulties as a challenge, as an opportunity to learn about yourself.

Learn how to deal with stress by paying attention to your breath, relaxing, not letting little things get to you. Let the little annoying things roll off your back, like a duck .

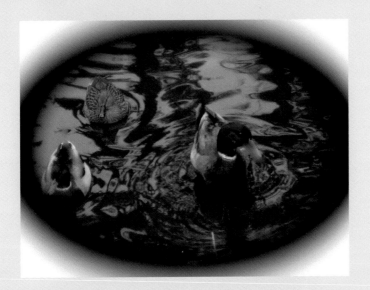

Be open to change, willing to learn, keep your curiosity about life

Be open to awe

Bathe your body in positive feelings

Search for opportunities to laugh

Believe in yourself

Three Pillars of Health

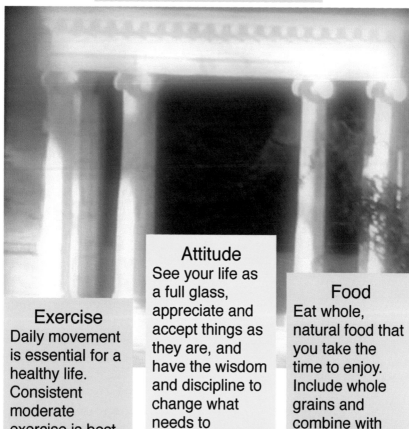

Exercise
Daily movement is essential for a healthy life. Consistent moderate exercise is best. Find something you enjoy doing and do it often. Good choices are:
- walking
- swimming
- biking
- skating
- yoga
- t'ai chi

Attitude
See your life as a full glass, appreciate and accept things as they are, and have the wisdom and discipline to change what needs to change. Allow yourself to be an imperfect human being, doing the best you can, and give yourself credit for the attempt. Look for the silver lining and walk on the sunny side of the street.

Food
Eat whole, natural food that you take the time to enjoy. Include whole grains and combine with beans for plant-based protein. Eat fresh fruits and vegetables. Avoid overly processed and deep-fried foods that contain trans-fats, or anything partially-hydrogenated.

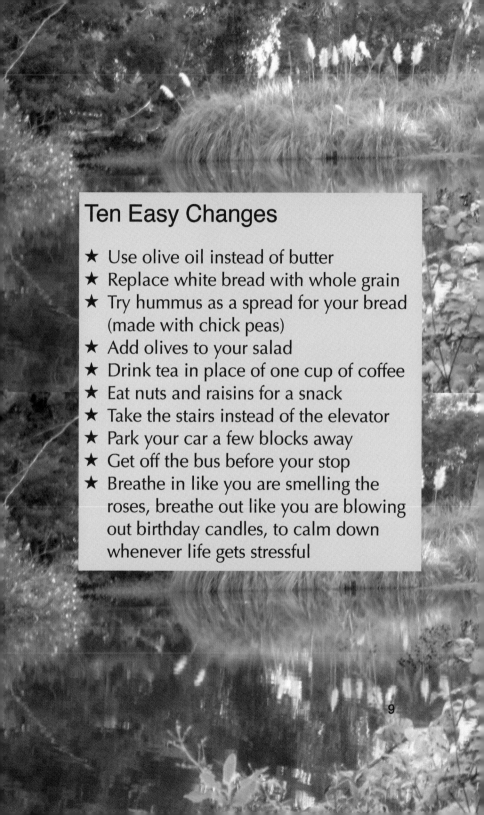

Ten Easy Changes

★ Use olive oil instead of butter
★ Replace white bread with whole grain
★ Try hummus as a spread for your bread
  (made with chick peas)
★ Add olives to your salad
★ Drink tea in place of one cup of coffee
★ Eat nuts and raisins for a snack
★ Take the stairs instead of the elevator
★ Park your car a few blocks away
★ Get off the bus before your stop
★ Breathe in like you are smelling the
  roses, breathe out like you are blowing
  out birthday candles, to calm down
  whenever life gets stressful

Relaxation

Belly breathing

Lie on a mat, on your back, knees bent, feet flat on the floor. Place your hands on your belly. As you breathe out slowly, feel your hands sink as your belly falls, and feel your hands rise as your belly fills with air as you inhale.

Breathe gently and easily, letting your exhalation become longer than the inhalation. You can count to 4 as you inhale and to 6 or 8 as you exhale. Let the exhalation become twice as long as the inhalation.

Relax and let the floor support you.

Key to relaxation: breathing

We don't spend enough time relaxing. We rush from the time the alarm clock goes off in the morning until we collapse, exhausted, in the evening. We need to spend more time consciously relaxing, so we can digest our food better, do cellular repair, let our heart rate come down, and allow our immune system to do its job of protecting us.

If we are always on - the go, then the sympathetic branch of our nervous system is in charge, and we can get worn down.

The parasympathetic branch takes over when we relax, when we rest and digest; slower heart rate, lower blood pressure, slower brainwaves and a feeling of peace can prevail.

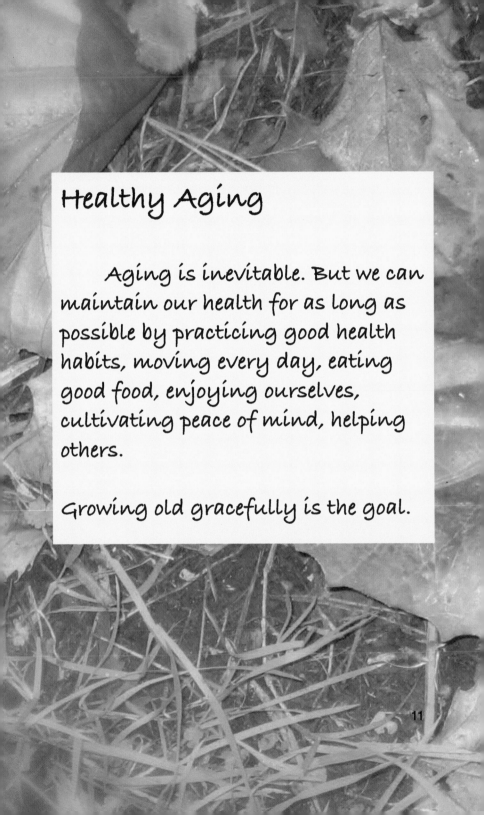

Healthy Aging

Aging is inevitable. But we can maintain our health for as long as possible by practicing good health habits, moving every day, eating good food, enjoying ourselves, cultivating peace of mind, helping others.

Growing old gracefully is the goal.

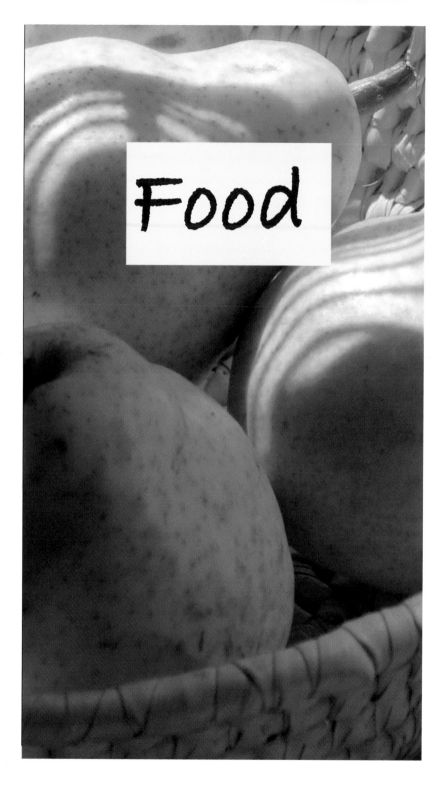

Food

How to Eat

The way the food news changes, it's hard to know how to eat. One day, butter isn't good for you, margarine is better, no wait, the trans fats are worse for you and butter is not that bad… Or low carb, high protein. Or is high carb, low fat better? No wonder people are confused!

Americans are consumed with losing weight, and yet obesity is one of our growing problems.

We feed grain to our livestock to fatten them up; but cows are ruminants and they are supposed to eat grass.

We have created foodstuffs that didn't exist 50 years ago. Chemically produced fats and sugars have confused our bodies, and have led to the insulin resistance, obesity and diabetes epidemic of Western culture.

Healthy Choices

Choose real unprocessed food

•fresh fruits
•vegetables
•whole grains
•heart-healthy fats
•fish
•nuts
•soy
•tea

Mindful eating

Take the time to savor what you are eating

Set the table

Put your fork down between bites

Eat smaller portions

Enjoy your food!

Healthy Populations

Okinawa is a series of 161 islands between Japan and Taiwan.

It may be the tropical paradise, eating the local varied vegetables and fish, the healthy amount of exercise built into daily life, the strong family bonds, the deep spiritual feeling, or all of these factors that account for the many centenarians living a long, healthy life.

Okinawans have the longest life expectancy, and the lowest rates of heart disease, stroke and cancer, which are the three main causes of death in the West.

We could learn from their example. One 95 year old says, "Eat good food (more fish, more vegetables, and less meat), walk everywhere and enjoy your work!"

Okinawan elders eat an average of 7 servings of vegetables and fruit a day, with 2 servings of flavonoid rich soy products per day.

They often have miso soup for breakfast (how different is that from bacon and eggs?). They have omega-3 rich fish several times per week and minimal dairy products and meat. They have very low rates of breast and prostate cancer, and they have strong bones in old age.

The oldest are considered national treasures, honored and included in society.

14

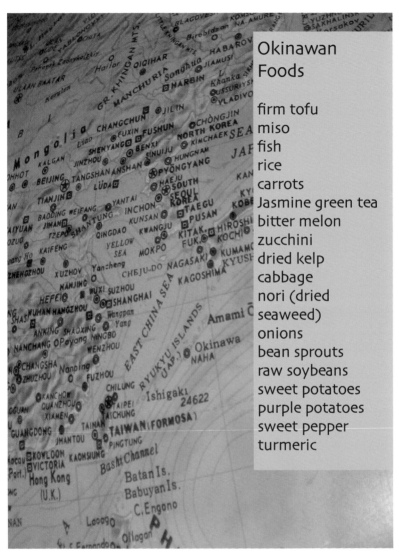

Okinawan Foods

firm tofu
miso
fish
rice
carrots
Jasmine green tea
bitter melon
zucchini
dried kelp
cabbage
nori (dried seaweed)
onions
bean sprouts
raw soybeans
sweet potatoes
purple potatoes
sweet pepper
turmeric

"Hari- Hatchi- Bu," eat until you are 80% full. It takes time for your stomach to tell your brain that you've had enough to eat.

Mediterranean region is noted for longevity and vitality

Mediterranean Foods

olives
olive oil
grapes
wine
tomatoes
tomato sauces
pasta
spinach
lettuce
carrots
whole grain bread
fish
garlic
onions
garbanzo beans

•Olive oil has been shown to lower LDL cholesterol, blood sugar levels and blood pressure

•Red wine has resveratrol, which has heart protective properties

Mediterranean Diet

Greeks and Southern Italians eat lots of olive oil, fresh fruits and vegetables, legumes, fish, bread, wine, and a small amount of dairy and meat. They do hard physical labor. They have close knit families and communities. They have low rates of heart disease.

French Paradox

In France, they eat a high-fat diet and their rates of heart disease are much lower than in the U.S. So how do the French do it? Maybe it's the wine with resveratrol, a powerful antioxidant.

The French are relaxed at meal time. They take three hours for lunch, savoring each bite, eating smaller portions of rich, but satisfying food, and enjoying each others company.

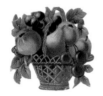

www.Mayoclinic.com

Healthy foods to include in any diet

garlic, onions—good germ fighters, antioxidants

carrots—beta-carotene, precursor of Vitamin A

blueberries, cranberries—high in antioxidants, good for bladder, kidneys

organic strawberries, oranges, peaches (in season)—high in vitamin C., fiber

walnuts—omega-3, good for healthy cholesterol, anti-Alzheimer's, good for ligaments, and joint health

almonds—calcium, magnesium, protein, fiber

sunflower seeds—high in the amino acid tryptophan, a precursor to the neurotransmitter serotonin. Eat a handful an hour before bedtime to promote sleep

black beans, aduki beans, white beans—high in fiber and protein

yogurt, kefir—good for intestinal flora

soy milk, tofu, miso—phytoestrogens, good for bone health, anti-cancer

cabbage, broccoli, cauliflower—anti-cancer

flax seeds, wild salmon—omega-3 essential fatty acids

olive oil—monounsaturated oil, good for heart health

whole wheat, barley, oats, bulgar wheat, millet, brown rice—good source of fiber and B vitamins.

tea—green, white, red, black—antioxidant

Weil, Andrew, MD. Healthy Aging

Essential Fatty Acids

Modern processed foods often contain **"partially hydrogenated"** vegetable oils that have extra hydrogen added to make a more stable molecule (like margarine). Unfortunately these become "trans-fatty acids" or **"trans-fats,"** which raise bad cholesterol, increasing the risk of coronary heart disease, even more than saturated fats. They also increase insulin resistance, which leads to diabetes.

Essential fatty acids are not produced by our body, so we need to get them from food. All of our cell membranes have a fat layer that is formed by the fats we eat. The cell membrane keeps the cell intact, and helps cells communicate with each other.

Fatty acids are chains of carbon atoms with hydrogen atoms attached to the side. If two hydrogen atoms are attached to each carbon atom in the chain, that is a "saturated fat." All of the available bonds are taken. This is a very stable compound, solid at room temperature (like butter). If the carbon atoms have double bonds with each other, then less hydrogen is present and these are "unsaturated," liquid at room temperature (like vegetable oil).

Monounsaturated fats have a single double-bond, like olive, canola, and peanut oils.

Polyunsaturated fats have two or more double carbon bonds like omega-3 and omega-6. Foods contain a mixture of these fatty acid types in varying proportions.

Good Fats vs Bad Fats

Good Fats

Omega-3
found in cold water fish
★salmon
★tuna
★sardines
★mackerel

★nuts and seeds
★flax seeds
★walnuts
★pumpkin seeds

Monounsaturated oils
★olive oil
★canola oil
★peanut oil

Bad Fats

Saturated Fats
(maybe not so bad)
found in animal products
•beef
•chicken
•full-fat dairy

Trans-fats
(really bad)
found in partially
hydrogenated vegetable
oil in processed foods
•margarine
•crackers
•cookies
•fast food

Wellness Molecule

Imagine if there were a substance that was a natural anti-inflammatory, that lowered blood pressure, helped joints maintain their flexibility, naturally improved your mood, and kept arteries flexible, especially the important coronary arteries that supply blood to the heart. It also improved skin texture and helped maintain blood sugar levels.

It would be a miracle drug, one that could improve the quality of everyone's life. There is such a thing, not a drug, but a naturally occurring substance, that our ancestors had more of in their diet than we have today. It's omega-3, an essential fatty acid, found in fish oil (yes, cod liver oil, our grandmothers were onto something!). It's an essential fatty acid, because our bodies don't make it, but we need it for healthy cell functioning.

How can it affect so many different areas in our bodies? Because it's found in all of our cell membranes and in brain cells as part of the neurotransmitter system of messaging between brain cells. It acts as a natural anti-inflammatory by mitigating the effects of inflammatory compounds produced by the immune system.

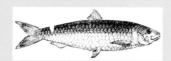

Omega-3 and Omega-6

There are two kinds of polyunsaturated fats: **omega-3 and omega-6**

They are very similar and compete for the same sites in your body, with different results. We need both, but the modern diet has about 20 times the ratio of omega-6 to omega-3. Our ancestors had more omega-3, found in wild game and foraged greens. Populations that consume a diet high in omega-3, like the Inuit, (Eskimos) have virtually no heart disease.

Omega-6 helps the immune system react to fight serious infection. It raises blood pressure slightly, and may contribute to heart disease by encouraging inflammation and helping blood to clot. Omega-6 is found in polyunsaturated vegetable oils like corn, sunflower and safflower.

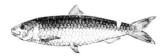

Omega-3

★anti-inflammatory

★blood thinner, reduces the risk of heart attacks and blood clots

★keeps immune system in check

★lowers blood pressure slightly

★improves mood

★reduces the pain of arthritis.

★found in cold water fish-
    salmon
    sardines
    mackerel
    tuna

★fish oil capsules are safe, as they have been purified of the heavy metals, which may contaminate fresh fish

★chickens fed fishmeal or flax produce eggs with omega-3

★flaxseeds and walnuts are good vegetarian sources

21

Anti-oxidants

Many kinds of compounds have antioxidant properties:

Flavonoids
responsible for the pigment (color) of fruits and vegetables:
•anti-inflammatory
•anti-microbial
•anti-cancer
properties

Isoflavones
kind of flavonoid found in soy and legumes

Polyphenols
tea
coffee
chocolate
berries

red wine has resveratrol

Oxidation is the interaction between oxygen and other substances. When you cut an apple it turns brown and when iron is exposed to air, it forms rust. Free radicals, which are unstable oxygen molecules that have one electron and are looking for another electron to complete its outer shell are responsible for the reaction.

In the body, oxygen will "borrow" an electron from a normal cell, which can damage cell membranes or DNA. Damage to DNA can lead to cancer.

Antioxidants can slow down the aging process, by keeping the cell from dividing more often. Antioxidants also protect against heart disease and cancer.

Foods highest in antioxidants

Fruits
blueberries
strawberries
raspberries
plums
oranges
red grapes
cherries
pomegranates
acai

Vegetables
kale
spinach
Brussel
sprouts
broccoli florets
beets
red bell pepper
yellow corn

Green Tea contains a powerful antioxidant, epigallocatechin gallate, (ECGC).
The more green tea you drink, the lower your risk of cancer and heart disease.

Lycopene, a powerful anti-oxidant found in red foods:
•watermelon
•guava
•papaya
•apricots
•pink grapefruit
• blood oranges
• tomatoes- more available in cooked, than raw tomatoes.

Beta-carotene—precursor of vitamin A (can be converted to Vit. A in your body) found in orange colored food:
•carrots
•sweet potatoes
•cantaloupe
•squash
•pumpkin
•apricots
•mangoes

Antioxidant compounds are more concentrated in the peel of the vegetable and the skin of the fruit. They protect the plant from microbes, viruses, and fungi.

Vitamins

Vitamins

Antioxidant Vitamins

Vitamin A (retinol) fat soluble, found in sweet potatoes, carrots, milk, egg yolks, cheese.

Vitamin C (ascorbic acid) water soluble, found in oranges, grapefruit, kiwi, strawberries, bell peppers.

Vitamin E (alpha-tocopherol) fat soluble, found in almonds, wheat germ, safflower, corn and soybean oil.

Vitamins

Vitamins are essential micronutrients found in food. They were discovered when sailors at sea, deprived of fresh foods, developed deficiencies like scurvy (lack of vitamin C) and beri-beri (lack of vitamin B).

The British Royal Navy found that lemons and limes cured scurvy during long sea voyages and they were known as "Limeys."

The Japanese Navy discovered that sailors eating only polished rice (white rice) developed beri-beri, which can lead to heart failure and weakness. Eating unpolished (whole brown) rice, reversed this B- vitamin deficiency.

Better to get vitamins from food, than in a bottle.

Fat Soluble Vitamins

•Vitamin A (retinol)
Found in butter, egg yolks, fish livers. Can be converted from beta-carotene, found in carrots, green and yellow vegetables.

Good for eyes, night vision,skin, resistance to infection.

•Vitamin D (cholecalciferol)
Manufactured in the skin in the presence of sunlight. Found in oily fish, fortified milk.

Helps absorption of calcium from intestines; essential for bone health.

•Vitamin E (alpha-tocopherol)
Found in wheat germ, seeds and beans.

Antioxidant. May be effective against heart disease and cancer.

Water Soluble Vitamins

•Vitamin B complex
Found in germ and bran of seeds, cereals, nuts, beans, liver, nutritional yeast.

Good for nervous system, anemia, depression.

•Vitamin C (ascorbic acid)
Found in citrus fruits, strawberries, bean sprouts, green pepper, sauerkraut.

Good for healing wounds, colds, inhibits histamine in allergic reactions. High doses can lead to kidney stones

Fat soluble vitamins can build up in your body, and too much over time in the form of supplements can be toxic.

Water soluble vitamins are nontoxic and any excess is excreted in urine.

Vitamin D

Effects of Vitamin D

★ promotes bone formation
★ regulates calcium and phosphorous levels in the blood
★ affects immune system
★ may prevent some cancers
★ may improve treatment of some cancers
★ may prevent or reverse heart disease

Food sources of Vitamin D

Fatty fish:
herring-3 oz =1383 IU
salmon-3.5 oz=360 IU
mackerel-3.5 oz=345 IU
sardines-1.75 oz=250 IU
tuna in oil- 3 oz=200 IU

egg= 20 IU

fortified milk, soy milk, breakfast cereal

IU=International Unit

Vitamin D isn't really a vitamin. It's a fat soluble substance discovered in 1920 by a British researcher who raised dogs in the wintertime without exposure to sunlight. He found that they developed rickets unless they were fed fish liver oil. In 1924, researchers found that exposing human skin to sunlight produces this "fat soluble vitamin," and as it was the 4th vitamin discovered, it was named, "Vitamin D."

It is actually a "pro-hormone", it acts like a hormone after it has been metabolized. In humans, vitamin D_3 (cholecalciferol) is converted from its basic building block (cholesterol) when ultraviolet- B (UVB) hits cells in the skin. After it is processed by the liver,and then the kidney, it becomes the fully active **calcitrol**. In plants, Vitamin D_2 (ergocalciferol) is converted from its basic building block (ergosterol) when UVB rays hit the leaves of the plant. Both forms can raise the amount of vitamin D circulating in the bloodstream.

Factors leading to Vitamin D deficiency

•Not enough exposure to sunlight, including:
    smog
    cloud cover
    northern latitude
    protective clothing
    sunscreen
• Melanin— the pigment in skin, makes it harder make sufficient Vitamin D
• Age—older folks have a harder time converting Vitamin D
• Obesity—makes it harder to absorb Vitamin D

Deficiency Diseases

•rickets (soft bones) in children
•osteomalacia (soft bones) in adults
•possible contributor to osteoporosis and gum disease
•associated with greater risk of depression, high blood pressure, cancer, auto-immune diseases

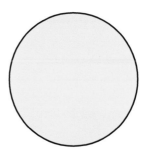

To produce adequate amounts of Vitamin D: 10-15 minutes of sun exposure without sunscreen to arms, legs or back at least 2x per week,when UV index is greater than 3

SPF 8 (sun protection factor) inhibits more than 95% of Vitamin D production in the skin

Recommended Daily Intake
400 IU for most adults
600 IU over 70 years old
UL (upper limit) 2,000 IU

New study recommends 1,700 IU

Increase in kidney stone risk with high dosage over time

http://www.ajcn.org/cgi/content/abstract/72/3/690

www.Wikipedia.com, Vitamin D

http://ods.od.nih.gov/factsheets/vitamind.asp

Benefits of fiber

* lowers LDL and triglycerides, thus lowering the risk of heart disease.
* stabilizes blood glucose levels by controlling insulin release by the pancreas and glycogen release by the liver.
* stimulates immune function by increasing production of T helper cells, antibodies, cytokines, and leukocytes.
* increases production of beneficial bacteria (probiotic)
* increases absorption of dietary minerals
* strengthens colon wall mucosa and inhibits adhesions.
* prevents constipation and diverticular disease

All plant foods contain soluble and insoluble fiber.

Insoluble fiber is found in the skin of fruits and vegetables and in whole grains like whole wheat and rye. Insoluble fiber provides bulk to stool, preventing constipation and diverticular disease.

Soluble fiber is found in the pulp of fruits like plums and berries, grains like oats and barley. Soluble fiber is fermented in the large intestine and yields short-chain fatty acids, which have several health benefits.

Insoluble fiber	Soluble fiber
whole grains bran (8g/cup) nuts(2-3 g/oz.) seeds	**legumes** lentils, peas, soybeans (15-19 g/c)
vegetables green beans, cauliflower (2-3 g/cup)	**grains** oats (4 g/cup) rye barley
fruits skins of some fruits, including tomatoes	**fruits** plums, berries, prune juice (7g/cup)
	vegetables Broccoli, carrots (2-3 g/cup) potatoes and sweet potatoes (4g/ half) psyllium seed husk (71g/ 100 grams)

American Dietetic Association (ADA) recommends 20-35 grams per day. Average American diet has 12-18g/day.

Fermented Foods

Many cultures around the world use fermented foods. Fermenting is an age old method of preserving food that converts sugar to lactic acid and in the process makes food more digestible.

Nutrients like essential amino acids and essential fatty acids are more available to us. The good bacteria like lactobacillus makes it harder for bad bacteria to grow.

Fermented foods contribute to good GI tract health. If you need to take antibiotics for a severe infection, make sure to repopulate the gut with probiotics, good bacteria like acidophilus found in yogurt after the course of antibiotics is finished.

yogurt, kefir, aged cheeses
(from milk)

wine, vinegar,
(from grapes)

olives

pickles
(from cucumbers)

sourdough bread

sauerkraut, kimchi
(pickled cabbage)

miso, tempeh
(from soybeans)

One centenarian said she couldn't live without her sauerkraut.

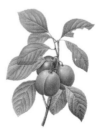

Benefits of Soy

Sources of soy protein

8 oz. soy milk =10 grams of soy protein

4 oz. of tofu =13 gr.

soy burger = 12 gr.

soy protein bar = 14

soy sausage =6 gr.

1/4 c. roasted soy nuts = 20 gr.

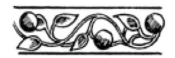

Soy may lower risk of:
★heart disease
★menopausal bone loss
★breast cancer
★prostate cancer
★osteoporosis

Soybeans have a plant-based protein containing all eight essential amino acids. They are high in protein and low in fat and cholesterol free. Soy contains isoflavones, which are phytoestrogens, a plant-based compound which is similar to estrogen, and can block estrogen receptors in certain tissues, possibly lowering the cancer stimulating effect of estrogen.

Soy also contains omega-3 fatty acids which help maintain healthy cell membranes. It has fiber, which maintains colon health, and has calcium, magnesium, and potassium for strong bones. It has B vitamins including folic acid for nerve health.

Soy Products

Tofu—bland cake in soft, silken, firm, and extra firm textures. Firmer tofu has less moisture and more protein and flavonoids.

Miso—fermented paste, salty, good for soup.

Tempeh—fermented cake.

Soy milk—creamy liquid made from soaked and cooked soybeans. Can be used in place of cows milk.

Soy flour—made of crushed soybeans, rich source of flavonoids.

Texturized soy protein dehydrated soy product. When rehydrated has texture like ground beef.

Soy nuts—roasted soybeans.

Edamame—boiled, salted young soybeans.

Some people are allergic to soy, and there are some conflicting studies about phytoestrogens and hormone disruption.

Highly processed soy foods may be harder to digest than traditional soy foods like tofu.

Fermented soy products like miso are generally easier to digest.

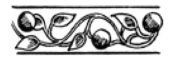

Women in Japan eat 30-50 grams per day of phytoestrogens. They have less trouble with hot flashes, less breast cancer and better bone density.

Benefits of Tea

All true tea is from the same plant, *Camellia sinensis.* The variations in tea come from different processing after it is picked.

White tea is not wilted or oxidized.

Green tea is wilted and not oxidized.

Oolong is bruised, wilted and partially oxidized.

Black tea is wilted, crushed and fully oxidized.

Black tea is heated while it is drying, to stop the oxidation process.

Tea has catechins, which are a kind of antioxidant. White tea and green tea have more catechins than black tea.

Tea contains theanine, an amino acid which can cross the blood brain barrier, and can elicit feelings of relaxation, reduce stress, improve cognition and mood when combined with caffeine.

Tea increases serotonin, dopamine and GABA, which are neurotransmitters in the brain.

Tea stimulates alpha brain waves, which are the alert yet relaxed brain waves.

Tea has been shown to improve immune response by boosting T-cells.

Caffeine Content
Tea has about 30—90 mg of caffeine, depending on how it brewed.

Black tea has about 50 mg/cup
Green tea about 15-30 mg/ cup.

Brewed coffee has 80—135 mg/ c
Drip coffee has 115—175 mg/ cup

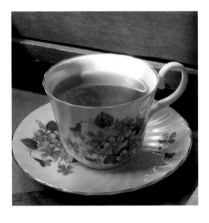

Green tea is best brewed with water under boiling temperature, (about 175° F.), for 30 seconds. Green tea has a unique antioxidant — epigallocatechin gallate, ECGC.

Matcha is finely ground green tea

*A study in Japan shows the more green tea consumed, 4-5 cups per day, the less heart disease, cancer, and overall mortality.

Rooibos- "Red Bush" tea from South Africa, has antioxidants, is low in tannin and no caffeine. A good choice for a before bed tea

Calcium

Calcium performs many important functions:
- ★Regulates permeability of the cell membrane, determining what flows in and out of the cell
- ★Affects the electrical potential of the cell, which controls muscle contraction and nerve function
- ★Controls blood vessel dilation and contraction
- ★Essential for glandular secretions, cellular communication, blood clotting
- ★Is a structural component of bones and teeth

The level of calcium in the blood is strictly controlled by hormones. If more calcium is needed, it's taken from storage in the bones.

Parathyroid hormone (PTH) draws calcium out of the bone to circulate in the blood.

Calcitonin, from the thyroid gland, directs calcium to be stored in the bone.

Magnesium suppresses PTH and stimulates calcitonin, which helps calcium to be stored in the bones.

Calcium absorption is partially blocked by oxalic acid (found in spinach and chocolate), and by phytic acid (found in raw beans, seeds, nuts, unleavened bread). Phytic acid is reduced by cooking, sprouting or fermentation. Probiotics can help with the digestion of phytic acid. Too much phosphorous (found in carbonated sodas) can decrease calcium absorption from the intestines.

Calcium is excreted when the diet is high in acid forming animal protein.

Vegetarians excrete less calcium.

Good Sources of calcium

Dairy Products
*8-oz part skim ricotta cheese = 509 mg
* 8 oz low fat yogurt = 415 mg
* 8-oz. non-fat milk = 306 mg
* 8-oz. whole milk = 276 mg
* 1-oz Swiss cheese = 224 mg

Fish
* 2 ounces of sardines with bones = 240 mg
* 3-oz canned pink salmon with bones = 181 mg

Legumes
1/4 block firm tofu = 163 mg
(prepared with calcium sulfate and magnesium chloride)
1 cup white beans = 191 mg
1 cup navy beans = 126

1 tbsp. blackstrap molasses = 172 mg
1 cup cooked beet greens = 164
1 cup cooked spinach = 245
1 slice cheese pizza =113
1/2 cup ice cream = 113
1 cup white rice = 111
1 cup cooked broccoli = 62 mg

Nuts
1 oz (24) almonds= 70 mg
1 tbsp. sesame seed tahini = 64 mg

USDA National Nutrient Database for Standard Reference, Release 17 Content of Selected Foods per Common Measure, sorted by nutrient content Calcium, Ca/ mg

Calcium needs magnesium and vitamin D to be absorbed. Your skin produces Vitamin D when exposed to sunlight for 10-15 minutes a day, without sunscreen.

Calcium supplements are better absorbed 500 mg. at a time. Chelated calcium is more bio-available. Calcium citrate is a good choice for a supplement.

Weight bearing exercise helps build strong bones:

Walking

Dancing

Running

Skating

Biking

T'ai Chi

Yoga

Climbing
Stairs

Exercise

Benefits of exercise

★ improve heart and lung function

★ increase metabolism

★ improve circulation

★ reduce cholesterol

★ increase bone mass to prevent fractures

★ improve mood

★ decrease depression

Any exercise
is better than
no exercise.

Ten minutes of
thinking about
exercise is better
than no exercise.

Ten minutes of exercising is
better than ten minutes of
thinking about exercising.

Exercising for 10 minutes 3 times
a week is better than 10 minutes
of exercise once a week.

Ten minutes of exercising 3 times a day
is better than ten minutes of exercising
3 times a week.

30 minutes of exercise every day is better
than 30 minutes of exercise 3 times a week.

Exercise is essential for a healthy life

Music can help add an extra bounce to your step.

What is the best exercise?

The best exercise is the one that you will do consistently. For most people that would be walking. You don't need any fancy equipment beyond a good pair of shoes and you can do it anywhere.

If you drive, you can park a distance away from your destination and walk. If you take the bus you can get off a few blocks before your stop. You can take the stairs instead of the elevator when practical. When you are shopping, you can park far away from the store entrance, and return the shopping cart to the front of the store, swinging your arms as you return to your car.

Rather than getting together with friends for coffee, take a walk together instead.

You can work walking into your day, everyday.

Try a meditative walk. Let your mind wander, and see what's on your mind. Pick one thing to focus on, something you are concerned about or planning. And then for an equal amount of time focus on feeling glad or grateful. And then finish your walk cultivating a feeling of peace.

Add more movement into your life. When you are folding the laundry, or doing the dishes, put on some music and dance!

Exercise Intensity

In the zone

Time spent exercising at a lower intensity can be beneficial. Just getting off the couch and going for a walk on a regular basis can help. Exercising often and consistently is better than exercising erratically at a higher intensity.

Aerobic exercise can help you burn fat by increasing fat-burning enzymes in your muscles. To exercise aerobically means to have your heart rate in the training zone, at 65%-80% of your maximum heart rate.

You can use the calculation of:

220 minus your age = maximum heart rate and figure 65-85% of that number.

Count your heartbeats for six seconds during exercise and multiply by 10 to figure out your heart rate.

Or if you are breathing deeply, naturally, able to talk, but not sing, you are in the zone. It may take a few minutes to get into the training zone, to raise your heart rate, and then you want to sustain the aerobic exercise for 12 minutes, minimum.

Aerobic Exercise
Walking briskly, swinging your arms, listening to upbeat music, around a track, or in a park is a fun way to exercise.

Bailey, Covert. The New Fit or Fat

Interval training

By increasing the intensity of exercise, for just a few minutes within your usual workout, you can increase your fitness level and your body's ability to utilize oxygen and burn fat.

Here's how: You warm up by walking at a moderate pace for 2-3 minutes, and then walk much faster or jog for 30 seconds, then go back to a moderate pace for two minutes and repeat for a 25 minute workout. On a scale of 1 to 10, 10 is full out exertion, moderate pace is 6; easy pace is 3.

Or can you can do five minutes of warm up, two minutes moderate pace and two minutes fast pace. Repeat slow-fast four times, and a three minute cool down.

Give yourself a day of rest between strenuous workouts, so your body can recuperate and rebuild.

Weight Training
Use it or lose it!

Adding weight training can help you build muscle, and muscle burns more calories, even at rest, than fat does. You lose muscle mass as you get older if you don't do anything, but you can increase your muscle mass at any age.

Good lifetime exercises:

walking

bike riding

dancing

swimming

skating

yoga

t'ai chi

41

Yoga

Different styles of yoga:

Hatha yoga—using only the body, medium paced, good for everyone, especially beginners.

Iyengar yoga—done with props like belts and small bricks. Emphasis on correct posture and holding the pose.

Viniyoga—focuses on the breath and chanting. Very gentle, good for people with chronic diseases.

Bikkram—hot room yoga—done in a room heated to over 100 degrees. Designed to raise your heart rate. Better for younger people.

Ashtanga—power yoga—vigorous, energizing, jumping from one posture to the next, more like a workout.

Flow yoga—poses flow into one another, more like dance.

Yoga is a gentle series of movements done with awareness and timed to the in-breath and out- breath, part of the ancient Ayurvedic system of medicine from India. It increases flexibility and strength; awareness of body and mind. There are standing poses, sitting poses and floor poses.

Breathing exercises can help you regulate your autonomic nervous system, which controls functions like digestion and heart rate. All of the poses are designed to prepare your body to sit still for meditation and ultimately for self-realization.

Everyone should own a yoga mat and spend a few minutes a day, at least, on the floor, rolling around and relaxing.

Get to know your own body

Here is one simple pose to get you started:

Savasana—Corpse Pose
(Deep Relaxation Pose)

Lie on your back on your yoga mat. Roll around for a few minutes to get comfortable.

Let your body sink into the floor. Close your eyes, breathe through your nose. Let your feet open to the side. Relax your arms at your sides, palms up. Relax your neck and jaw. Let your mouth open slightly, but continue to breathe through your nose. Just notice your breath, no need to control it. Imagine your limbs feeling heavier as you relax into the floor. Let your eyelids relax.

Stay in this position for 5 minutes as a beginner. To maintain the feeling of relaxation, come out it slowly, roll onto your side and push up with your hands to a seated position. This is usually done at the end of a yoga class, but can be beneficial at the end of a workday, for a few minutes of relaxation.

It is best to learn yoga from a qualified instructor.

T'ai Chi

T'ai Chi is an ancient form of movement from China. It is a "soft" martial art. The slow dance-like movements are performed with awareness of the breath. It is a form of "moving meditation."

T'ai chi is especially good for the joints and for maintaining balance and coordination for older people. By practicing tai chi you can calm your mind and increase your chi (life force).

Qigong (chi kung) is a movement system from China, designed to raise and store your chi. Incorporating standing postures with very deliberate shifting of body weight from one foot to the other. It is more static than tai chi. Good for increasing healing energy.

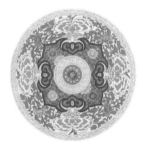

http://nccam.nih.gov/health/taichi/

chi exercise

Stand with your feet shoulder width apart, knees soft, slightly bent, not locked. Hands at your sides, palms facing back.

Tuck your tailbone slightly under, as if there were a weight attached to the sacrum (bottom of the spine).

Imagine a string at the top of your head, lifting your head toward the sky.

Tuck your chin slightly.

Let your belly be soft, as you breath deeply, letting the abdomen fill with each breath, and empty with each exhale.

As you inhale, let your wrists rise up, as if there were a string attached to them, elbows sinking, lifting only your wrists.

Leave your shoulders down and let your fingers be limp.

As you exhale, let your arms flow down, wrists leading, fingers following, back to your sides.

Repeat three times.

Feel your chi (life force) gathering in your lower abdomen (dan tien) below your navel.

Pilates

Six principles of Pilates

1. Centering—bringing the focus to the center of the body.
2. Concentration—full attention and concentration to the exercise for maximum benefit.
3. Control—every exercise done with complete muscular control.
4. Precision—awareness sustained throughout each movement.
5. Breath—very full breath, using the lungs as bellows to strongly pump air fully in and out during exercise.
6. Flow—fluidity, grace, and ease are the goals of exercise carried into every day life.

Joseph Pilates was a German stage performer who was forced into internment in England during WWI. He developed a series of exercises done with precision and concentration on the breath to strengthen the core muscles of the abdomen.

Pilates is done on a mat or on special equipment that he designed from bed springs to provide resistance. The movements are done slowly, with control and an emphasis on the proper form, not repetitions, to develop elongated muscles and graceful posture.

http://pilates.about.com/od/whatispilates/a/WhatIsPilates.htm

Sample Pilates Exercise

"The Hundred"

Lie on your back, on a mat, and bend your knees, feet flat on the floor.

Have your lower back in a neutral position, not arched or tucked.

Bring your knees halfway to your chest, and raise your head towards your knees.

Your hands rise up a few inches off the floor and flap them, while your abdomen is scooped.

Breathe in deeply through your nose and then exhale through your mouth as you count to ten.

Repeat the breathing and hold the position until you reach 100 (ten full breaths).

http://www.videojug.com/film/pilates-how-to-achieve-great-abdominals

Sleep

Lack of Sleep

inhibits ability to concentrate

increases pain perception

increases depression

decreases immune response

magnifies the effects of alcohol, causing impairment

slower reaction time when driving, similar to being intoxicated

sleep debt- you can get less than optimum sleep for a few days, and then make it up.

sleep deficit- but chronic sleep debt leads to poor health

How much sleep do you need?

Sleep is an important aspect of a healthy life. During sleep your body repairs and regenerates bone and muscle and strengthens the immune system. It's a prime way we cope with stress, solve problems, and recover from illness.

People vary in how much sleep they need by age, activity level, and body type. Infants need 16-18 hours a day of sleep. Teenagers on average need 9 hours, and most adults need 7-8 hours of sleep. When you wake up and feel well rested, that's how much sleep you need.

We are becoming a sleep deprived culture. With so many distractions to keep us up late, (the TV, computer, movies, cell phones etc.) colliding with the necessity to get up early, most of us are not getting the good deep sleep that we need.

http://harvardmagazine.com/2005/07/deep-into-sleep.html

Sleep cycles

stage 1—(Drowsiness) 5 or 10 minutes-easily awakened.

stage 2—(Light sleep) heart rate slows, body temperature decreases.

stages 3 & 4—(deep sleep) difficult to awaken. Blood flow decreases to the brain, redirects toward muscles. Immune function increases.

REM (rapid eye movement) (dream sleep) occurs about 70-90 minutes into your sleep cycle. You have 3-5 REM episodes per night. Breathing is rapid, irregular and shallow, heart rate increases, blood pressure rises.
REM sleep is essential for processing emotions, memories and stress.
Better REM sleep improves mood and memory.

If you are sleep deprived, REM sleep is made up first.

Sleep deprivation and obesity
insulin sensitivity and appetite-related hormones are affected by lack of sleep.

Leptin is a hormone related to appetite control.

Ghrelin is a hormone that is an appetite stimulant.

Lack of sleep causes leptin levels to fall and ghrelin levels to rise.

Tired people are hungrier, more apt to eat out of control.

Insomnia

Studies show that people who sleep 6.5 hours to 7.5 hours a night live the longest.

If you are not sleeping, don't worry about it. Just rest quietly.

Power resting can be almost as good as sleep.

Keep your bedroom as dark as possible.

Melatonin, a hormone secreted by the pineal gland, paves the way for sleep.

Light inhibits melatonin.

A lousy nights' sleep makes you feel miserable. What can be done?

Start with your mind—what is worrying you so, that you can't sleep? Can you make a date with yourself to worry about it later? If not, get up and write about it. At least you won't have to worry about forgetting it.

Or did you have too much caffeine too late in the day? You can fix yourself a cup of warm milk with honey,and a banana, or sunflower seeds which are high in tryptophan, to give yourself the precursors of the neurotransmitter serotonin that helps you relax and drift off to sleep.

You can't *make* yourself go to sleep; you can only allow yourself to surrender to sleep.

Persistent insomnia can be a symptom of an underlying condition like depression. See your doctor.

Progressive relaxation

Contract and then relax your your muscles slowly, one by one, starting at your toes, working your way up your legs and then each arm. Contract and relax the muscles of your face. Let all of your muscles relax, feel heavy and exhale through your mouth.

Breathing

Count backwards from ten, breathing out slowly and deeply, letting each breath get slower and deeper. Let your belly rise and fall with each breath. If you get all the way to one, start again. By giving your mind something to focus on, and utilizing your breath which is the link between the voluntary and involuntary parts of your nervous system, you can gain control of your body and mind.

To help you sleep

★Write down what's troubling you

★Arrange a time for worry

★Eat a handful of sunflower seeds which are high in tryptophan, one hour before you want to go to sleep

★Breathe slowly, deeply, counting down from 10, letting each breath get slower and deeper. When you get to one, start from ten again

★Just rest, imagine sleep is a swinging door, that you are waiting to enter

★Pretend that you are asleep

Self massage

One area that needs to relax before you can drift off to sleep is the back of your neck. With our culture's emphasis on the visual—reading, computers, TV, etc,— we have lots of eyestrain. The optic nerve exits the spine at C2, (the second cervical vertebra), near the top of the neck.

Place both hands on the back of the neck, and rub firm little circles along the ridge of your skull, (occipital ridge) especially the two bumps at the base of your head (occiput). Work down your neck with one hand squeezing the muscles with your fingertips along one side of your neck. Switch hands and work the other side.

Small movements can help relax your neck too. While lying in bed, tuck your chin slightly with each exhalation, and raise your chin slightly with each inhalation. You can count down from 10 to 1 while doing this, and make each exhalation longer and slower than the one before. Try a sigh of relief (a long deep slow exhalation with the "ha" sound after each set of ten breaths.) Then pretend you're drifting off to sleep.....ahhh...

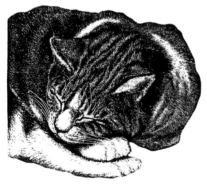

Sleep Hygiene

Get up and go to bed at the same time every day

Take naps before 3 p.m.

Exercise vigorously, but not within 4 hours of bedtime

Have a light snack before bed, eat all heavy meals at least 4 hours before bedtime

Avoid caffeine after 4 p.m.

Use your bed only for sleep (and sex)

Make your bedroom dark and a little cool

Practice the same sleep rituals, brushing teeth, washing face, etc, so your body knows it's time to go to sleep

Take a hot bath 90 minutes before bedtime. It's your body cooling down that sends the message to the brain that it's time for sleep

When you feel your body start to cool down, when you get the urge to go to sleep, follow it. Sleep comes in cycles. Catch the wave....

Visualization

Pretend that you are gently falling, like floating downward with a parachute.

Imagine little green men in orange jumpsuits with toothbrushes scouring all your joints from your feet up, with bubbling foam until your whole body is filled with a white foam. Then imagine a silver shower starting in your head and rinsing your whole body clean. Feel that all your limbs are so heavy that you can't possibly move them. This heaviness is what happens when you fall asleep.

Imagine a beautiful ice skater dressed in white, skating around in a circle in your minds eye. Hear the sound of the ice-skating blade gliding over the ice. The lulling monotony of white on white and going around in a circle will lull you to sleep.

See what you can visualize that works for you

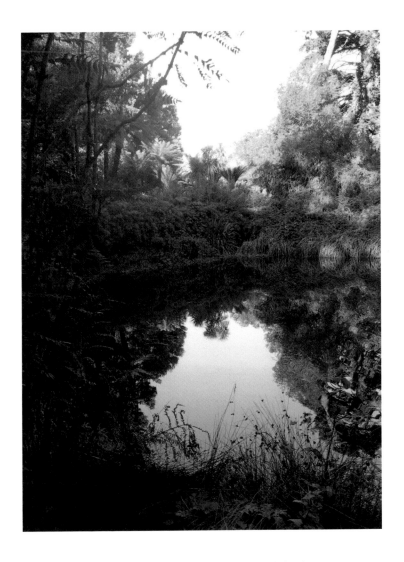

Imagine yourself in a totally peaceful place.
Smell the flowers, hear the birdsong, feel the
gentle breeze on your cheek.

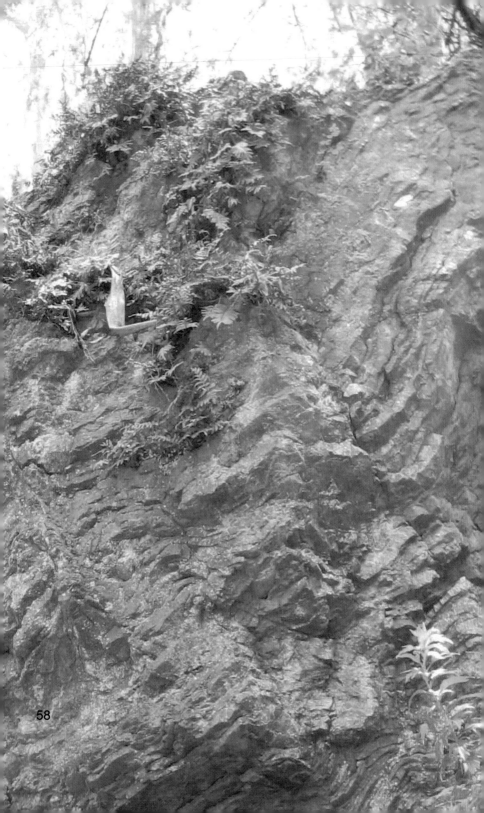

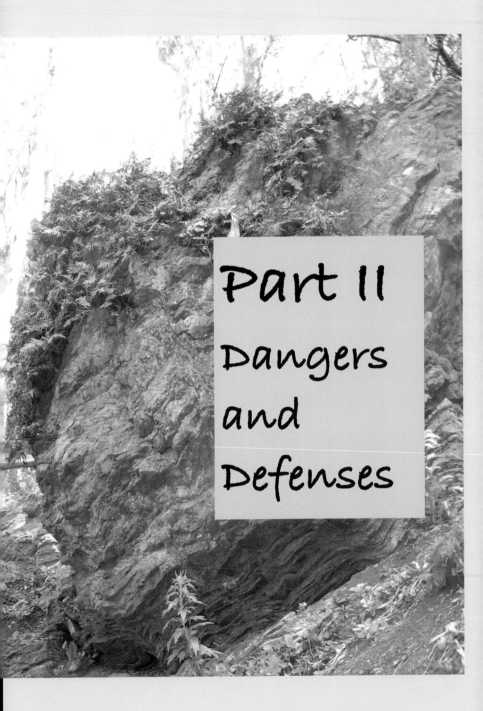

Part II
Dangers
and
Defenses

Stress Response

Imagine it's after midnight and you hear a noise at your front door, awakening you out of a light sleep. Your heart starts racing, blood pressure rises, your breathing is shallow, and your palms are sweating. Blood is directed away from the gut and digestion, to the large muscles of your legs in preparation for fight or flight. The sympathetic nervous system is in charge.

Now imagine the same stimulus, the same noise at your front door, but this time you have a teenager who has just learned how to drive. Now your reaction is different, you breathe a sigh of relief, your heart slows down, blood pressure drops, palms are dry. The parasympathetic branch of the nervous system takes over, digestion resumes, cellular repair occurs, sleep is deeper.

The stimulus, the noise is the same, but your reaction is totally different. Stress is not something that happens outside of yourself. *It is your own response that makes something stressful.* It is your perception of reality, your interpretation of events.

stress breakdown

1. stressor—the outside event or stimulus
2. your interpretation of the stimulus
3. your physiological reaction

You cannot eliminate stress from your life, but you can become aware of it and learn different ways to respond

Breathe

60

Physiology of the stress response

Your stress response is geared to respond to acute physical danger. Your blood is shunted to your legs for a quick get away. Your heart beats faster, blood pressure rises, and blood sugar surges to fuel the large muscles. Digestion and cellular repair is put off until later. Reproduction is put on hold until a more opportune time.

All of these responses are okay for short term emergencies, but can be damaging to your body if they go on too long. During times of chronic stress, blood pressure is elevated,and the stickiness of the platelets increases, which can cause atherosclerosis (hardening of the arteries). Plaque can build up which can decrease blood flow and increase the risk of heart attacks.

If everyday life is an emergency, then the stress response can wear your body down

Stress cannot be avoided in modern life, but we can learn to respond differently, to change the way we interpret stimuli, to calm down by using our breath

The nervous system

Voluntary   Autonomic

         /   \

sympathetic—parasympathetic

Our nervous system responds to the world around us and inside of us. The nervous system has two parts. The voluntary branch, which directs your muscles to move, and an autonomic branch that controls heart rate, blood flow, digestion, things generally not under our conscious control.

The autonomic system has two branches, the sympathetic and the parasympathetic. Like the gas and brakes of a car, they work in tandem, one inhibiting the other. The sympathetic is like the gas, the get-going branch. It directs the blood flow to the large muscles of the legs in flight or fight situations. Some of these nerve endings are in the adrenal glands (above the kidneys), which releases adrenaline (also known as epinephrine). The parasympathetic controls digestion, cellular repair, sleep, and growth. The parasympathetic is the dominant system when you are relaxed, acting as a brake to the sympathetic branch.

relax

Hormonal response to stress

hypothalamus-pituitary-adrenal connection
(H-P-A axis)

The brain activates the stress response. The hypothalamus, which responds to emotions, secretes corticotrophin releasing hormone (CRH) which directs the pituitary gland to secrete adrenocorticotropic hormone (ACTH), a hormone signaling the adrenal gland to produce glucocorticoids, which are steroid hormones like cortisol. These hormones are released when something stressful happens, or even *when you think stressful thoughts.*

Glucocorticoids raise blood pressure, and inhibit immune system response. Production of growth hormone is inhibited. Along with ACTH, the pituitary gland produces other hormones like prolactin, which suppresses reproduction.

Epinephrine, from the sympathetic nervous system, is released quickly and acts quickly, while glucocorticoids act over a period of minutes or hours. Excessive glucocorticoids contribute to fatigue, type 2 diabetes, hypertension, osteoporosis, premature aging and death.

Sapolsky, Robert Why Zebras Don't Get Ulcers

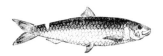

Endorphins, a natural pain killer are produced under severe stress; that explains why soldiers on the battlefield have an altered perception of pain.

After salmon spawn, they have high levels of glucocorticoids in their system. They have huge adrenal glands, peptic ulcers, and collapsed immune systems. If their adrenal glands are removed, they can live for another year.

Stress, Inflammation and Heart Disease

Heart disease is the leading cause of death in the United States. Stress and inflammation both play a part in heart health.

One type of cholesterol, low density lipoprotein, is a fat and protein molecule that settles out of the bloodstream and is deposited on the coronary artery walls, which supply blood to the heart. Your body makes a cap over this deposit called a plaque, which narrows the space for blood flow, that can lead to higher blood pressure.

Inflammation can cause the cap to disintegrate, leading to the cap dissolving and clotting agents being released, and then you can have a heart attack.

Inflammation is a part of your body's defense system; it's the way we combat germs with specialized white blood cells. Even an infection elsewhere in the body, like gum disease, can play a part in heart disease.

You can measure the level of inflammation in your body with a test called C- reactive protein or CRP.

• raising your blood pressure, making it more likely for the cap to burst.
• directing blood to flow to limbs, not organs, thereby postponing digestion and decreasing the liver's ability to process cholesterol
• putting off cellular healing and repair, when your body might have been able to fix it

Heart health

Heart disease

Heart disease is the number one killer in the United States today. It affects roughly one hundred million people, about half of the population. Clearly the typical American diet contributes to the prevalence of this disease.

The Honolulu Heart Program Study started in 1965 to compare three different populations from Japan. One group living in Japan, eating primarily vegetables, rice, fish, soy and a little meat, with a group of Japanese living in Hawaii eating a mixture of Japanese food and American food (milk and hamburgers), and a group residing in Los Angeles eating a totally Americanized diet. The first group had very little heart disease, the second group had some and the third group had more.

There are genetic risk factors for heart disease, and there are modifiable lifestyle factors. Part of understanding your own risk for heart disease is understanding cholesterol and what those numbers mean, and understanding blood pressure, and what that indicates about your health.

http://www.stanford.edu/group/ethnoger/japanese.html

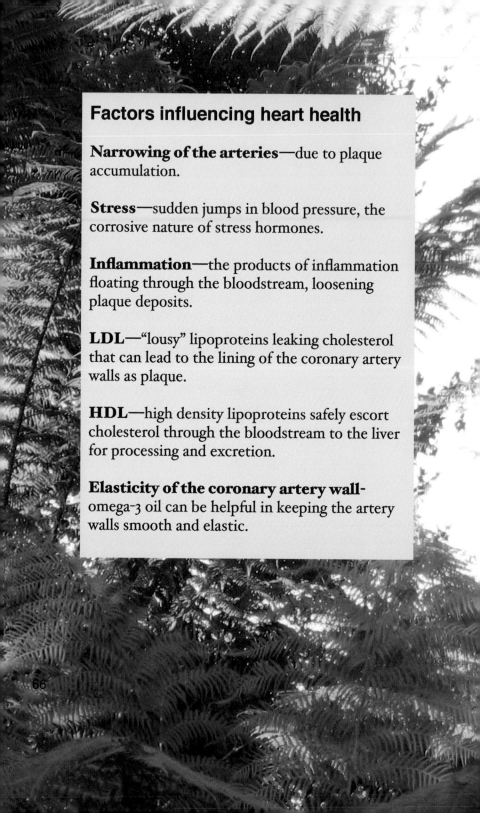

Factors influencing heart health

Narrowing of the arteries—due to plaque accumulation.

Stress—sudden jumps in blood pressure, the corrosive nature of stress hormones.

Inflammation—the products of inflammation floating through the bloodstream, loosening plaque deposits.

LDL—"lousy" lipoproteins leaking cholesterol that can lead to the lining of the coronary artery walls as plaque.

HDL—high density lipoproteins safely escort cholesterol through the bloodstream to the liver for processing and excretion.

Elasticity of the coronary artery wall-omega-3 oil can be helpful in keeping the artery walls smooth and elastic.

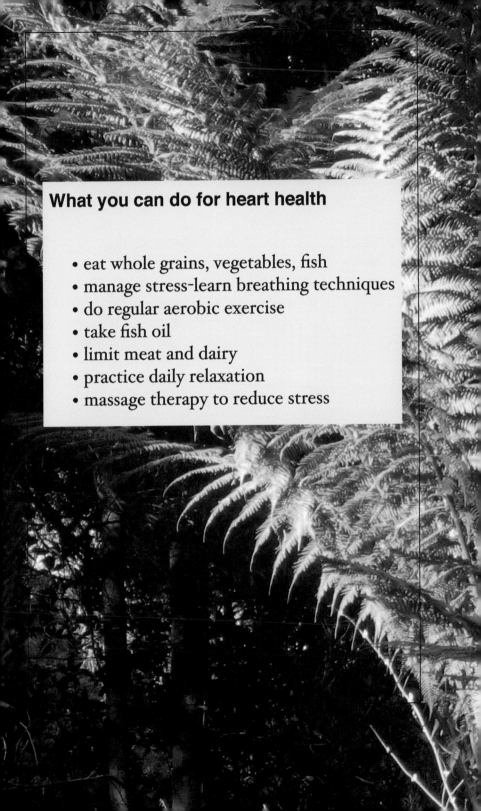

What you can do for heart health

- eat whole grains, vegetables, fish
- manage stress-learn breathing techniques
- do regular aerobic exercise
- take fish oil
- limit meat and dairy
- practice daily relaxation
- massage therapy to reduce stress

What is Cholesterol?

Cholesterol is a naturally occurring soft waxy substance found in all cells, and is used to form cell membranes, certain hormones (chemical messengers) and some tissues. It is produced by the liver and is also found in saturated animal fats. It is a lipid (fat) which cannot be dissolved in the bloodstream, which is mostly water, so it attaches to a protein to produce a lipoprotein (fat and protein molecule) for transportation through the body.

High Density Lipoproteins (HDL) are made up of mostly protein and very little fat, forming a stable package and the cholesterol it carries does not deposit on the artery walls. It can scavenge LDL and carry the cholesterol back to the liver, where it can be processed and excreted.

HDL averages about 25% of total cholesterol. A high level of HDL, over 60, is considered heart protective. A low level HDL reading is below 40 for men and 45 for women. Average levels are 45 for men and 55 for women. Estrogen tends to raise HDL, so as women enter menopause, HDL levels drop.

Low Density Lipoproteins (LDL) are made up of fat and a little protein, forming an unstable package that can deposit cholesterol along coronary arteries, contributing to heart disease.

An optimal level of LDL is below 100. A reading of 160 is high.

The size of the LDL particles can be predictive of heart disease. The smaller, denser particles are more likely to block arteries. An advanced lipid test can screen for these particles, which are genetically determined.

68

Piscatella & Franklin. Take A Load Off Your Heart

Two kinds of Lipoprotein:

High Density Lipoprotein
(HDL)
High levels of HDL are protective

Low Density Lipoprotein
High levels of LDL are destructive
(LDL)

Fats that raise your HDL -
(Hooray!—the way to remember it —
the good kind)
(monounsaturated)
olive ,canola, peanut oil
and
(polyunsaturated) fish oil

Fats that raise your LDL
(Lousy—the way to remember it)
(saturated) animal fat
and
*partially hydrogenated
vegetable oils*
also known as "trans-fats"

Cholesterol Counts

Total cholesterol should be
under 200

200-239 borderline high

240 and above-high

LDL—below 100
160 high risk

HDL—60 and above,
Below 40—high risk

HDL ratio- to LDL
should be below 3.5

High blood pressure is called **hypertension**, and it can get steadily worse over the years, increasing your risk of heart attack or stroke.

Dizzy spells, chest pain, swelling in ankles and feet, headaches, changes in vision or concentration could be a sign of hypertension.

Healthy blood pressure is *120 and below over 80 and below.*

Pre-hypertension is *120-139 over 80-89.*

Stage one hypertension is *140-159 over 90-99.*

Stage two hypertension is *more than 160 over more than 100.*

Blood pressure

Blood pressure measures how your heart contracts and relaxes, pumping blood through your body. Any resistance, either a narrowing of the artery wall, due to deposits, or a loss of elasticity will increase blood pressure.

Blood pressure is measured in two parts. The first number. (the *top number*) is called the *systolic* pressure and this is a measurement of how strongly the heart contracts to push a volume of blood through the heart. The second number (the *bottom number*) is called *diastolic* pressure and this is a measurement of the heart relaxing, between beats.

Blood pressure varies throughout the day, and especially with stress. Some people have "white coat hypertension" meaning their blood pressure goes up when the doctor takes it. You can take your blood pressure three different times and average them to get a true picture of your blood pressure, if you are borderline high.

Triglycerides

Calories which are not used immediately are converted to triglycerides and transported to fat cells. Hormones regulate the release of triglycerides from the fat cells so your body's energy needs are met between meals.

Elevated triglycerides can indicate coronary heart disease, even when cholesterol numbers are low. Triglycerides are measured by a blood test and the results are the number of milligrams in a deciliter of blood.

Normal- less than 150 mg/dl
Very high- 500 mg/dl and up

To bring down triglyceride levels:

eat less
exercise more

cut back on sugar, simple carbohydrates, alcohol

increase fish, fiber, complex carbohydrates

eat breakfast
don't eat late at night

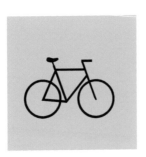

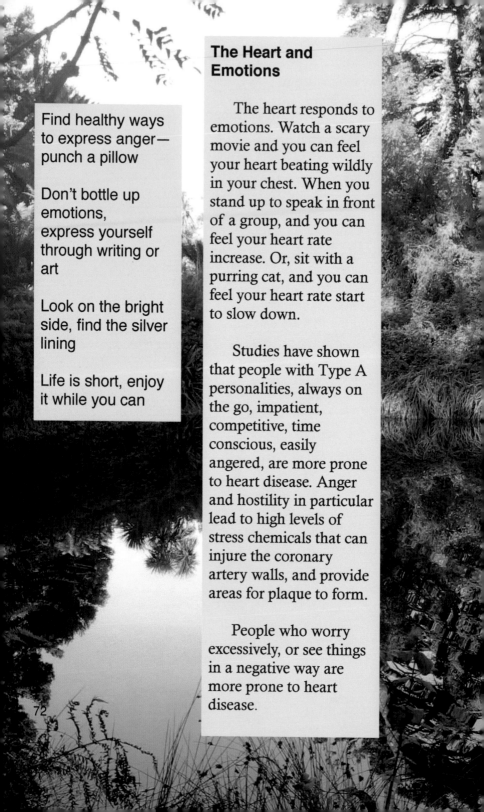

Find healthy ways to express anger— punch a pillow

Don't bottle up emotions, express yourself through writing or art

Look on the bright side, find the silver lining

Life is short, enjoy it while you can

The Heart and Emotions

The heart responds to emotions. Watch a scary movie and you can feel your heart beating wildly in your chest. When you stand up to speak in front of a group, and you can feel your heart rate increase. Or, sit with a purring cat, and you can feel your heart rate start to slow down.

Studies have shown that people with Type A personalities, always on the go, impatient, competitive, time conscious, easily angered, are more prone to heart disease. Anger and hostility in particular lead to high levels of stress chemicals that can injure the coronary artery walls, and provide areas for plaque to form.

People who worry excessively, or see things in a negative way are more prone to heart disease.

72

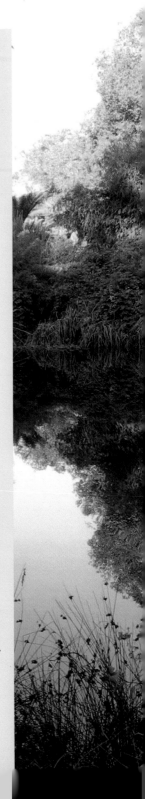

Loving Kindness Meditation

Sit comfortably in a quiet place. Let your breathing slow and deepen. Think of someone that you love, a friend, a lover, a parent or a pet. Feel your heart opening and filling with loving kindness as you think of this person. Now think of someone else, someone perhaps you have some difficulty with. See if you can send this person that feeling of loving kindness that you just generated. Now imagine someone whom you feel is your enemy. See if you can send that person some lovingkindness in the spirit of compassion and forgiveness.

Now turn that feeling of lovingkindness toward yourself. Feel your heart open in acceptance and love for yourself. Give yourself the same compassion and forgiveness that you gave to others.

Thondup, Tulku. The Healing Power of Mind

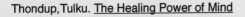

Immune System

White blood cells have different jobs; some sound the alarm, some surround and engulf the enemy, some attack tumors, and some tell the body when the fight is over and it's time to clean up the damage.

Lymph fluids travel throughout the body, but lymph doesn't have a pump. It relies on pressure gradient differences produced by breathing and muscular contraction.

When you move, you move the lymph around. When you move you create more cellular waste products.

Massage therapy is a unique opportunity to move the lymph without you moving and creating more cellular waste products.

Your immune system protects you from foreign invaders—bacteria, viruses, fungi, toxins. When it operates properly, it recognizes what is "you" and what is not you.

White blood cells, the primary cells of the immune system, are found in the lymph system, which closely follows the blood circulation.

The lymph system is made up of the tonsils, the thymus gland, the spleen, lymphatic vessels, and lymph nodes. Lymph carries water and protein back to the blood and clears away cellular waste products. Lymph is found in the small intestine, in the interstitial fluid, (the fluid surrounding cells), in lymph vessels, and is filtered in the lymph nodes.

The lymph of the head and right arm drain into the right lymphatic duct; the rest of the body drains into the thoracic duct. Both ducts drain into the circulatory system at the subclavian vein, underneath your collar bone.

Inflammation is the way your body deals with injury or infection. The area gets red, hot, swollen, and hard to move. Initially, small blood vessels in the immediate area become dilated and blood flow slows down. Blood vessels become leaky, permitting passage of water, salts, and small proteins into the interstitial space (the space between the blood cells). White blood cells head to the scene. Macrophages, a kind of white blood cell, surround and engulf any bacteria present.

Inflammation is a process of building up and breaking down tissue. The proteins for tissue repair are present and the white blood cells, which devour bacteria and other foreign substances, are active. In acute inflammation, this is very helpful. In chronic inflammation like arthritis, the body can devour surrounding tissue. In cases of auto-immune dysfunction, the body can destroy healthy tissue, mistaking itself for a foreign invader.

Chronic inflammation is a marker for heart disease, cancer, and diabetes. Eating natural anti-inflammatory foods like fish oil may decrease your risk for these diseases.

Your body has an amazing capacity to heal itself. What happened to that annoying paper cut you had last week?

Types and Amounts of White Blood Cells

- neutrophils   40 - 75 %
- eosinophils   5 %
- basophils   0.5 %
- monocytes   1 - 5 %
- lymphocytes   20 - 50 %

Neutrophils are the most abundant type of white blood cell and the first to respond to infection. They are short lived, with only a 12 hour life cycle. They engage in phagocytosis, which is a process of engulfing bacteria and destroying them with enzymes. They die soon after phagocytosis and are the major component of pus.

Eosinophils are found in allergic reactions. They have surface receptors for the antibody **immunoglobulin E (IgE)**. They increase in the mucosal lining of the nose and bronchial tubes during hay fever and asthma. The count is highest in the morning and lowest in the afternoon.
IgE may be involved with the body's defense against cancer.

Basophils and **mast cells** have very specific receptors for **IgE** produced in response to various allergens. They produce histamines and in the most serious cases, anaphylactic shock.

Monocytes are the largest white blood cell and can live the longest. They can leave the bloodstream and become tissue macrophages.

Lymphocytes are the most numerous white blood cells in children and the second most numerous in older children and adults. They increase in response to viral infections. B-lymphocytes are formed in the bone marrow and T-lymphocytes are also formed in the bone marrow, but they are stored and brought to maturity in the thymus gland.

Kinds of T-cells

Helper T-cell:once activated, they rapidly divide, and secrete "cytokines" chemical messengers between cells that regulate immune response.

Cytotoxic T cells: destroy virally infected cells, tumor cells, and which are involved with transplant rejection.
.
Memory T cells:persist long term after infection, help body remember past infections. May be either CD4+(T-helper/inducer) or CD8+(T- suppressor/ cytotoxic).

Regulatory T cells: suppress immune response after event is over.

Natural killer T cells: (CD 161) special kind of lymphocyte that bridges the adaptive immune system with the innate immune system.

Almost every thing living has an innate immune system, which responds to threats in a generalized way. The adaptive immune system, found in vertebrates, recognizes and remembers previous infections and mounts a specialized response with B-cells and T-cells.

www.Wikipedia.com/immune system

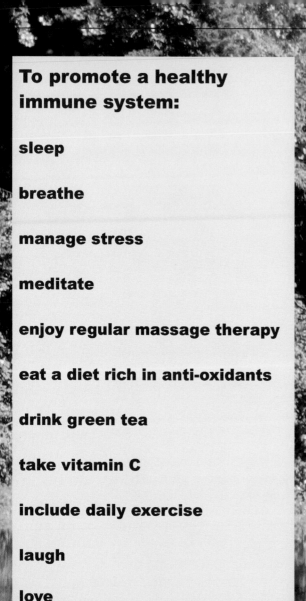

To promote a healthy immune system:

sleep

breathe

manage stress

meditate

enjoy regular massage therapy

eat a diet rich in anti-oxidants

drink green tea

take vitamin C

include daily exercise

laugh

love

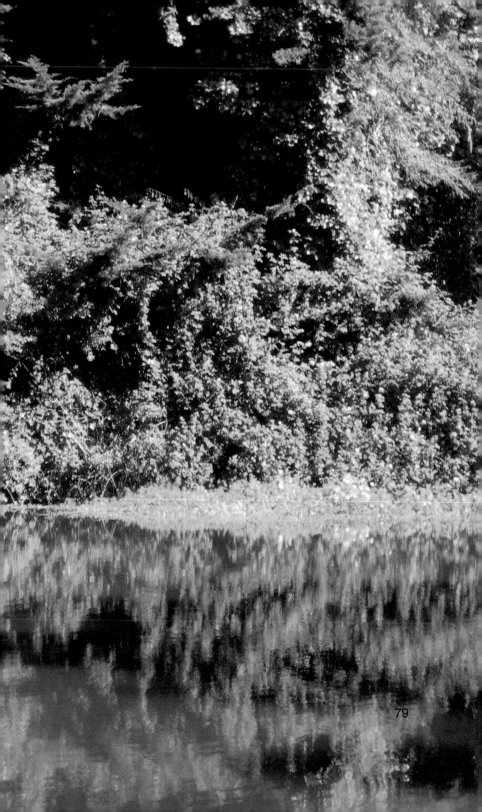

Illnesses

Risk factors:
- age—men over 40, women over 50
- high blood pressure
- high triglycerides
- high LDL
- low HDL
- obesity
- chronic kidney disease
- diabetes
- excessive alcohol,
- drug abuse, e.g. cocaine
- cigarette smoking
- chronic high stress

Classic symptoms of heart attack:
- sudden chest pain
- pain radiating to the left arm or left side of neck
- shortness of breath
- nausea
- vomiting
- palpitations
- sweating
- anxiety
- chest pressure
- feeling of impending doom

Heart attack

Heart attacks are the leading cause of death for both men and women all over the world. Known as myocardial infarction, it occurs when the blood supply to the heart is interrupted. When the coronary arteries which supply the blood to the heart are blocked due to the rupture of plaque, (an unstable accumulation of cholesterol and white blood cells), the resulting restriction of blood supply to the heart (ischemia), and oxygen shortage, if not treated, can result in damage to the heart or death.

Women may experience fewer classic symptoms, most often:
- shortness of breath
- weakness
- a feeling of indigestion
- fatigue.

If you experience one or more of these symptoms
Call 911 immediately

Cancer

Cancer is the second leading cause of death in the U.S.

Cancer is really a hundred different diseases with one thing in common —cells reproducing, out of control.

All cells in the body grow, divide, multiply and die. Cancer cells either keep multiplying out of control or they don't die off when they should. Something has happened to the genes (DNA) inside these cells that tells them what to do. There may be something inherited that potentially triggers these cells to become cancerous, or/and something in the environment makes the cells turn cancerous. Cells that divide often are more susceptible to cancer, like skin, bone, digestive tract, lungs. Damage to DNA adds up over time, so people living longer are more likely to get cancers.

www.cancer.gov

·Sulforaphane is a compound found in cruciferous vegetables like
·broccoli
·cabbage
·cauliflower
· kale
·brussel sprouts, which has been shown to inhibit cancer.

Broccoli sprouts have the most sulforaphane.

Vitamin D is protective against the development of cancer

Green Tea has anti-cancer properties

Stress management can help improve the functioning of the immune system.

Signs of cancer

- persistent cough
- persistent swollen glands
- blood tinged saliva
- change in bowel habits
- blood in stool
- unexplained anemia
- lump in breast or testicles
- change in urination
- blood in urine
- change in wart or mole
- unexpected weight loss, night sweats or fever
- non healing sores
- all of these signs can have non-cancer causes

As we understand the mechanisms of cancer better, the treatments will get better.

The kind of gene that allows a cancer to form is called an oncogene. The cell changes (mutates) and starts multiplying rapidly. It can form a mass of cancerous cells (tumors). Tumors can secrete enzymes that protect them from immune system attack. Tumors can create their own blood supply. Cancer cells can travel to other sites in the body through the blood or lymph system (metastasis).

We may have cancerous cells in our body all the time, but our immune cells are looking for them. Tumor suppressor genes stop tumors from forming. There are natural killer cells in the immune system that root out cancerous cells and kill them.

http://www.emedicinehealth.com/cancer_symptoms/page2_em.htm

Stroke

Stroke is the third leading cause of death after heart disease and cancer. A stroke is a medical emergency, also known as a brain attack.

There are two kinds of stroke, the more common one is called **ischemic**, when a blood clot forms in a blood vessel in the brain.

The other kind is **hemorrhagic**, when a blood vessel breaks and there is bleeding in the brain.

Transient ischemic attacks, or TIAs, are very brief episodes of the blood not circulating properly. These can indicate a greater likelihood of a major stroke at a later date.

There is a medical treatment, tPA, (tissue plasminogen activator) effective for 3 hours after an ischemic stroke. This would not be used when there is bleeding in the brain.

http://www.stroke.org/

Signs of stroke:
sudden numbness on one or both sides, hands or feet or face

sudden confusion and the inability to speak or understand language

sudden loss of vision in one or both eyes

sudden loss of balance, difficulty walking

sudden intense headache

If you experience one or more of these symptoms **Call 911 immediately**

Risk factors for stroke:
similar to heart disease

Keeping blood pressure down is the best way to prevent strokes.

83

Signs of diabetes:

•increased urination

•increased thirst

•increased appetite

•weight loss

•blurred vision

•ketoacidosis, the smell of acetone on the breath.

Diabetic complications:

•doubles the risk of cardiovascular disease

•kidney failure, requiring dialysis

•blindness

•poor wound healing, especially on the feet, possibly leading to amputation

Diabetes can be diagnosed with a blood test, by measuring blood sugar levels.

A random plasma glucose reading of 200 mg/dL or a fasting glucose reading of 126 mg /dL or above indicates diabetes.

Diabetes

All cells need glucose for fuel. Glucose can't get into the cell directly; it needs insulin to act as a key to open the cell membrane to let the glucose in. The pancreas produces insulin.

Some people lack the ability to make insulin. They have type 1 diabetes, and need to inject insulin. Other people make some insulin, but not enough, or their cells are not sensitive enough to insulin. These people have Type 2 diabetes.

Type 2 diabetes used to be called adult onset, but many children are being diagnosed with it now, so it's called Type 2 diabetes. The incidence of Type 2 diabetes is increasing with the obesity epidemic of the last 20 years, in the U.S. About 20 million people have been diagnosed with diabetes, 8% of the population, and about 57 million have "pre-diabetes" and don't know it.

www.diabetes.org

Certain populations seem to have a genetic predisposition to diabetes: African-Americans, Hispanics, Asian Americans, Pacific Islanders, and Native Americans. They may have inherited a "thrifty gene" from the past when they experienced feast or famine. Today the main factor is obesity. The more you eat, the more insulin you need to get the glucose into your cells. The more overweight you are, the more resistant to insulin you become, and the more insulin you need. If you don't have enough insulin, then the level of glucose in your bloodstream rises.

The body's preferred fuel is carbohydrates, which convert to glucose most readily. If no carbohydrates are available then the body utilizes its fat stores.

But what leads to insulin resistance in the cells? One prime suspect is trans fats, from partially hydrogenated oils. Trans fats interfere with proper functioning of the cell membrane. It could be the key to keeping insulin out of the cell. It is widespread in the typical American diet, especially in fast food. Combined with super-sized sodas full of high-fructose corn syrup, these could be the cause of the obesity and diabetes epidemic.

Type 2 diabetes can be managed with lifestyle changes

Properly timed **exercise:**to lower the glucose in your bloodstream, brisk walking is sufficient

Diet:high in **fiber, fruits and vegetables,** low in saturated fat and sugar

stress reduction: stress causes blood sugar to rise —liver releases stored glucose to deal with emergencies

Chemicals to avoid

Bisphemol A (BPA)—
found in plastic lining of
metal cans and in plastic
containers labeled #7
*Buy tomato sauce in
glass jars instead of cans
*Buy powdered baby
formula instead of in
cans
*Use glass baby bottles
instead of plastic

Teflon—breaks down at
high temperatures and
leaches toxic chemicals
*Use cast iron instead

Phthalates—softens
plastics, lowers sperm
counts

PBDE—flame retardant
similar to PCB and DDT
Thyroid hormone
disruption and possible
carcinogen

Pesticides—nerve
toxins
*Buy organic produce
whenever possible

Environmental Illness

Thousands of
chemicals are in our
modern environment, and
we are absorbing them in
the food we eat and the air
we breathe.

Some of the chemicals
that go into making plastic
are similar to estrogen and
can become hormone
disrupters, contributing to
the risk of reproductive
cancers.

Air pollution,
especially diesel exhaust
can contribute to
respiratory diseases like
asthma. Living near a
freeway can put
communities at risk.

Neurotoxins like lead,
mercury, pesticides, PCB
(fire retardant) may
contribute to the increased
incidence of autism and
ADHD (attention-deficit-
hyperactivity-disorder).
Infants and children are
more susceptible to the
effects of chemicals, due to
their smaller size and rapid
development.

Environmental Working Group http://www.ewg.org/
National Institute of Environmental Health Sciences National
Institutes of Health http://www.niehs.nih.gov

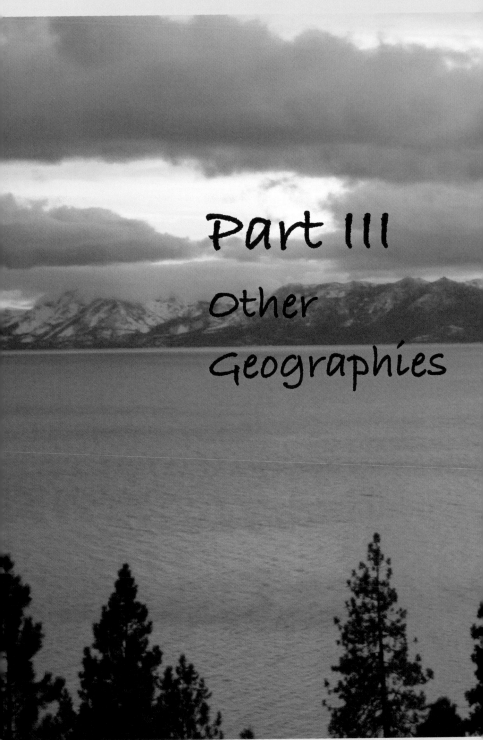

Part III

Other Geographies

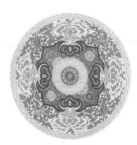

Chinese Medicine

The history of Chinese Medicine in the West
In the 1970's President Nixon opened up relations with China, which had been closed to the West since 1949. The first delegation of westerners included James Reston, a reporter for the NY Times. He had an appendectomy in China and experienced first hand, acupuncture for post surgery pain relief.

Chinese Medicine has been evolving for 5,000 years. It is based upon observing nature, and how the forces of nature are repeated in the human body. By paying close attention to the way energy waxes and wanes throughout the day, and how the change of season affects health, Chinese Medicine practitioners are able to keep their patients well.

In the old days in China the doctor was paid to keep you healthy. If you got sick, he wasn't doing his job well, so payment stopped. This idea of health is closer to ecology or organic gardening. It's better to keep someone healthy than to treat them after they get sick. Better to keep the immune system strong, so a person is more robust, able to handle stress, than to nurse them back to health after an illness.

Other Geographies

Bill Moyers in his groundbreaking TV series **Healing and the Mind** says " there are other geographies of the body, other maps that guide healers in other cultures."

Chinese Medicine, in which the body is viewed as an energy system, seeks to restore the harmonious flow of chi and balance the opposing qualities of yin and yang. Chi is the vital life force in every living being.

Chinese Medicine modalities include acupuncture, herbs, massage, movement, (t'ai chi) and concentration (Qigong). The patient is responsible for maintaining their own health through physical movement and meditative balance.

The Chinese Medicine practitioner tries to determine whether chi is flowing or stagnate and if yin or yang is excessive or deficient. The five-element theory further delineates weaknesses and strengths of one's constitution. The eight guiding principles help determine disharmonies of the moment.

Some illnesses are due to "pernicious external influence," like being exposed to a cold draft, or toxic substances. Herbs can help strengthen the person's immunity.

Chi (Qi)

Chi is the vital life force that defines everything that is alive. Original chi (wu chi) is the chi that we are born with, that we inherit from our parents. What we do with that chi, whether we husband it, or squander it, depends on our lifestyle. Some people have stronger chi to start out with, and can party the night away without ill effects, while others have to watch more carefully, how they spend their energy.

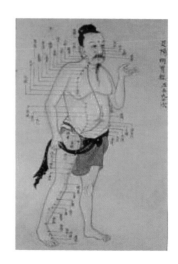

We derive chi from the foods that we eat and the air that we breathe. Chi flows through the acupuncture meridians, energy channels throughout the body. The flow varies throughout the body, depending on the time of day, like the tides in the ocean. We have stronger chi when we are younger, and it diminishes as we age, unless we strengthen it with exercises like t'ai chi or qigong.

Yin and Yang

Yin and *yang*, are the two interdependent forces of nature found everywhere. Everything has its own opposite, and one cannot exist without the other. Darkness exists in relation to light. Male and female, hot and cold, day and night. Happiness does not exist without the idea of sorrow.

The *yin organs* are the solid organs, deeper in the body, which store chi.

•lungs
•heart
•pericardium
•liver
•kidneys
•spleen

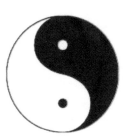

The *yang organs* are the hollow organs, closer to the surface, which conduct chi.

•large intestine
•small intestine
•gallbladder
•bladder
•stomach

Night doesn't cause day;these opposites exist in relationship to each other, and each contains a bit of the other.

Five-Element Theory

The world is formed by five elements--Wood, Fire, Earth, Metal, and Water. These elements or forces are in relationship to one another. There are two cycles of relationship, one nurturing or giving rise to, the other constraining or controlling. They are sometimes described as similar to mother and child relationships. The meridians are named for organ functions, like Lung (breathing) or Stomach (digesting), not anatomical locations. Chi flows through different meridians, depending on the time of day.
        (see chart)

Nurturing cycle,

Water nourishes Wood

Wood feeds Fire

Fire generates Earth

Earth creates Metal

Metal enhances Water

Controlling cycle:

Wood controls Earth

Earth contains Water

Water controls Fire

Fire constrains Metal

Metal controls Wood

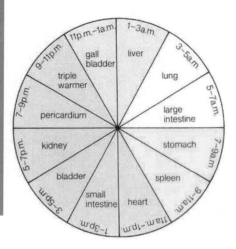

Five element theory correspondences

Element	Wood	Fire	Earth	Water	Metal
Direction	East	South	Center	North	West
Time-of-Day	Dawn	Midday	Afternoon	Midnight	Dusk
Sleep-State	Waking	Wakeful-ness	Transition	Slumber	Quiet
Season	Spring	Summer	Late Summer	Winter	Autumn
Yin Organs	Liver	Heart	Spleen	Kidney	Lung
Yang Organs	Gallbladder	Sm. Intestine	Stomach	Bladder	Lg. Intestine

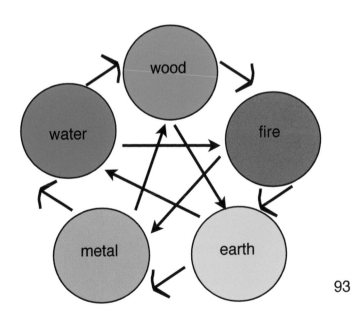

93

Eight Guiding Principles

Cold: Slow metabolic activity, sensations of cold or chill, low body temperature, pallid complexion

Heat: Increased metabolic activity, sensations of heat or burning, increase in body temperature, reddening or flushing of complexion

Deficiency: Low capacity or function of an organ system and low resistance to stress or infection; feelings of fatigue, weakness, emptiness or dull pain

Excess: Hyper functioning or obstruction of organ system and excessive reactivity to stress or infection; feelings of fullness, tension, agitation or intense pain

Internal: Affects deeper levels of the body, including visceral organs, brain, spinal cord, bones, nerves, middle and inner ear internal reproductive organs

External: Affects superficial layers including skin, hair, nails, peripheral vessels, nerves, muscles, tendons, ligaments, joints, eyes, external ears, nose, mouth, teeth, external genital organs

Yin: Composite nature of disease process that includes cold, deficiency, and internal syndromes

Yang: Composite nature of disease process that includes heat, excess, and external syndromes

If you are agitated or anxious, try drinking strong mint tea, it has a cooling effect. Other cooling foods are cucumber and tofu.

If you are cold and lethargic, try adding ginger to warm chicken soup.

What to Expect from a Chinese Medicine Practitioner

Diagnosis

Chinese medicine uses direct observation of you, the patient, to make a diagnosis.

The practitioner will look at your complexion, note the vitality in your eyes, notice any smells, as clues to the state of your health.

She may ask you questions about your sleep, diet, elimination, menstruation, injury, stress, and family health.

Pulse diagnosis

The practitioner will take your pulse, using three fingers and checking at three different depths, thus taking nine pulse readings on each wrist. The description of the pulse will be something like wiry or stringy, weak, strong, slippery, dry. Each quality reflects the state of energy in each meridian.

Tongue diagnosis

The practitioner will also look at your tongue, noticing if there is a whitish coat of mucous, if the tongue has ridges on the edges, if the tongue is jumpy while being held out for examination. The ridges or cracks down the center will also be noted, as these reflect on the inner state of the body.

Chinese Medicine is like organic gardening. You are like a healthy plant strengthened from within to avoid falling ill. By using Five Element theory, to determine your constitution; tonifying chi where deficient, and dispersing excessive chi, using such modalities as herbs and acupuncture.

Treatment

Putting together the pulse and the tongue reading, your practitioner will devise an acupuncture treatment, prescribe a combination of herbs, or he may suggest a meal plan, perhaps soups or teas to nourish.

Acupuncture is a treatment that adjusts the energy flow in the body. Slender needles are used on points along the meridians to simulate or sedate chi. The chi may be blocked, stagnant or excessive. An acupuncture needle is a little thicker than a strand of hair, and is placed just under the skin. It can feel like a little pinch, but nowhere near as painful as a hypodermic needle. Sometimes the acupuncturist will twirl the needle to generate a stronger response. No one really knows how acupuncture works, but it seems to stimulate the body's own healing mechanisms. It also produces a mild euphoria. It has been very effective in helping drug addicts with withdrawal. In China it is used as anesthetic during surgery. It can be helpful for all kinds of musculoskeletal pain, swelling, digestive disturbances, and allergies.

Moxibustion is a treatment for warmth or deficiency. A lit stick of mugwort is held over acupuncture points.

Cupping is a treatment that uses vacuum suction in glass globes for muscle injury, congestion, headache, and joint pain.

Massage therapy, called Tui-na, uses the hands and fingers to direct the flow of chi throughout the acupuncture meridians of body. Somewhat more vigorous than Swedish massage, utilizing skin rolling techniques, Tuina addresses musculo-skeletal and other soft tissue conditions.

Chinese herbs are given in combination, in individualized formulas. Like adding nutrients to the soil of a garden, they are a potent form of medicine to build up the constitution of an individual.

Chinese Medicine and Western Medicine

Chinese medicine:

Concerned with relationships, seeing the body as a whole.

Seeks to balance qualities such as heat or dryness, excess moisture or cold.

Like gardening, adding nutrients here, trimming excess energy there.

Health is a dynamic balance, always changing. The emotions change, the chi moves.

Chi is stuck or it's not flowing or it's deficient or excessive. Health is all about the balance of chi.

The doctor is seen as a teacher or a guide to help you maintain your own health. In the old days the doctor was paid as long as you stayed healthy. If you became sick, you didn't pay him, because he had failed to prevent the illnesses before it became manifest.

Good for chronic, or vague, pain, and discomfort. Can be helpful for infertility, and complementary cancer care.

Western medicine:

Depends on cause and effect. Take this drug and it will have this effect.

Like a garage mechanic, fixing this leaky pipe here, adding this fuel additive there. No accounting for the emotional state, unless working with mental illness.

Pay our doctors when we see them, when we are already ill. They hold our high esteem and we hope they have the magic bullet to cure us. We don't feel ultimately responsible for our own health. This attitude may be changing, and indeed has to change as our chronic diseases respond best to lifestyle changes, not necessarily to drugs and surgery.

Good for trauma, infectious disease, and emergencies.

97

Ayurveda

Ayurveda is the ancient art and science of daily living for health and longevity from India. Understanding each person's unique body, mind, and consciousness, is the foundation of health and happiness. Ayurveda is translated as "the science of life" from two Sanskrit words, "ayus" meaning life and "veda" which is knowledge or science.

The purpose of Ayurveda, according to Deepak Chopra, "... is to tell us how our lives can be influenced, shaped, extended, and ultimately controlled without interference from sickness or old age. The guiding principle of Ayurveda is that the mind exerts the deepest influence on the body, and freedom from sickness depends on contacting our own awareness, bringing it into balance, and then extending that balance to the body. This state of balanced awareness, more than any kind of physical immunity, creates a higher state of health."

Chopra, Deepak. <u>Perfect Health</u>

Ayurveda treats the whole person, seeking the underlying causes of disease, not just treatment of the outer symptoms.

Ayurveda originates from the 10,000 year old Vedas, which are revelations from meditative sages, transmitted through generations in an oral tradition, passed down in small phrases or poetry known as sutras.

"That person who always eats wholesome food, enjoys a regular lifestyle, remains unattached to the objects of the senses, gives and forgives, loves truth, and serves others, is without disease"
(Vagbhata Sutrasthana)

Like a seed that contains the whole of a tree, the sutras are a microcosm of wisdom.

The purpose of life, according to Ayurveda, is to realize cosmic consciousness, in one's daily life. The health of the physical body is important, as a means to experience divine consciousness.

Five elements

*Prana, the basic principle of the *air* element, is the flow of Consciousness from one cell to another in the form of intelligence. It is the vital life force necessary for all movement within each cell and throughout the whole body. Involuntary movements of heart, respiration, and peristalsis are governed by prana.

*Akasha is *ether,* all pervading, omnipotent, omniscient, omnipresent, pure spiritual energy. Expansive, empty, it has no resistance, and has freedom in which to move. It is the first expression of consciousness, the basic need of the bodily cells.

Agni, the basic principle of the *fire* element, is the transformative principle. It governs the metabolic processes regulating the transformation of food into energy; digestion, absorption and assimilation. Responsible for body temperature, agni is carried by the blood throughout the body. Poor circulation causes cold hands and feet. Fire regulates understanding, comprehension, selectivity and can be found in the body as the flame of attention.

Apas, the *water* element, is associated with chemical energy. Water is the universal solvent, governing all biochemical functions. The plasma in our blood is 90% water, and carries nutrients throughout the body. Together with the lymphatic system this is the Water of Life.

Pruthivi, the *earth* element is hard, dense, and solid. Bones, cartilage, nails, teeth, and hair are made up of earth element. It cradles and holds all living creatures, provides food and shelter.

All the elements are present in everyone but in individual proportions.

Health is a balance of all the elements.

Out of balance, diseases can occur.

Too much earth element results in obesity or depression.

Too much water can lead to edema.

Too much fire can lead to fever, inflammation, heartburn, anger or hate.

Prakruti

Everyone is born with a unique constitution or "prakruti", made up of five elements:
  Ether or Space
  Air
  Fire
  Water
  Earth

These five elements form the three doshas, or body types:

  Ether and Air
  form Vata,

  Fire and Water
  form Pitta

  Water and Earth
  form Kapha.

The three types correspond roughly to the ectomorph (thin build), mesomorph (medium build), and endomorph (sturdy build) in the West. Everyone has some of all three doshas, their own unique balance, though one or two doshas are usually prominent.

Tri-dosha

Vata controls movement. The body type is usually thin frame and has difficulty gaining weight., The vata type is prone to anxiety, insomnia,and erratic sleeping and eating patterns.

Pitta controls metabolism. The body type is medium build and moderate weight. They tend to be focused, organized, punctual, and perfectionist. They have red or blond hair, freckles, get angry easily, and they don't like hot weather.

Kapha controls structure. This body type tends toward a heavy build with dark thick wavy hair. They are slow, relaxed, calm, hard to wake in the morning, have slow digestion, and are slow to get angry. They tend to procrastinate and are predisposed to obesity, high cholesterol, allergies, sinus and respiratory problems.

	Vata	Pitta	Kapha
Frame	thin	medium	stout
Weight	low	moderate	heavy
Complexion	dull	ruddy	pale
Skin	thin, dry	warm, moist	thick, soft
Hair	scanty, coarse	moderate, fine, early grey	thick, wavy

103

According to Dr. Vasant Lad, Professor of Ayurveda,

"The three doshas, acting together, govern all of the body's metabolic activities. *Kapha* promotes anabolic activities, which include growth and the creation of new cells as well as cell repair. *Pitta* regulates metabolism by governing digestion and absorption. *Vata* triggers the catabolic process that is necessary for breaking down larger molecules into smaller ones. Since vata is the principle of movement, it acts on both pitta and kapha , which are both otherwise immobile.

Therefore when vata is out of balance, it influences and disturbs the other doshas, which is why the majority of all illnesses have aggravated vata at their source."

> Modern life could easily be classified as vata out of balance; moving fast and filled with anxiety.

Lad, Vasant. Textbook of Ayurveda

The doshic balance is dynamic. The time of day, the time of year, the time of your life, all play a part in determining the proper balancing of the doshas of each individual. Each person, each energy system, is unique. Some people can stay up late studying and function well the next day, some people can't. Some people pop out of bed in the morning, some people can't. By better understanding our own unique makeup, we can honor our own constitutions, and limits, and try to form our habits to strengthen our weaknesses and recognize our strengths.

Basic ayurvedic healing principles are that like increases like and opposites decrease each other. If one has too much heat, which is a pitta imbalance, then a cool drink or cooling herbs will help, rather than hot or spicy foods, which increases pitta. "Pitta governs not only our physical metabolism, but also the way we process, or digest, every outside impression that we encounter," according to Dr. Lad. "Thus, when in balance, pitta promotes intelligence and understanding and is crucial for learning. But when pitta is out of balance it can arouse the fiery emotions, such as anger, hatred, criticism, and jealousy."

Ayurveda divides our life span into three parts.

Birth to 16 is *kapha* when the body is forming and growing

16-50 is *pitta*, an age of activity and vitality.

Beyond 50 is *vata*, when the catabolic breakdown processes are apparent.

105

Six Tastes

The doshas are influenced by the six tastes:

Sweet (sugar and starches): building and strengthening, in excess can damage spleen and pancreas

Salty (table salt / seaweed): softening, laxative, sedative, in small amounts stimulates digestion, in excess can damage the kidneys

Sour (fermented food / acid fruit): stimulant, carminative (dispels gas), in excess can damage the liver

Pungent (hot spices like cayenne pepper or ginger): stimulant, diaphoretic (promotes sweating), improves metabolism, in excess can damage the lungs

Bitter (herbs like goldenseal / gentian): cleansing, detoxifying, in excess can damage the heart

Astringent (tannins, herbs like red raspberry, / witch hazel): stops bleeding and other discharges, promotes healing of skin and mucous membranes, in excess can damage the colon

'*Agni*' is digestive fire. Toxins or undigested food or waste is called '*Ama*'. Ama forms when agni is low. Ama conditions contribute to allergies, arthritis, and cancer, and can weaken the immune system, leading to metabolic imbalance, and auto-immune syndromes.

Detoxification is an important part of Ayurvedic therapy. *Pancha Karma* is a clinical practice of detoxifying and should be done under supervision of a trained Ayurvedic practitioner.

Ayurveda is good for many common aliments such as: allergies, asthma, backaches, respiratory ailments, gastrointestinal disorder, hypertension, PMS, stress, depression, chronic fatigue, and cardiovascular disease. An ayurvedic practitioner will design a custom made treatment plan based on physical examination of your pulse, tongue, eyes, face, lips, nails, urine, and an extensive questionnaire of your lifestyle habits to determine your dosha balance.

Methods of balancing the doshas include:

- color therapy
- sound or music therapy
- chanting
- gemstones
- yoga asanas (postures)
- pranayama (breathing exercises)
- meditation
- massage therapy
- correct diet for your dosha

Being mindful of everything that we take in through our senses has an effect on energy fields that influence our health. Whatever we do on a daily basis for ourselves, will have a greater effect than what someone else does for us. Daily and seasonal routines can prevent or correct imbalances before they lead to poor health. We can take control of our actions (karma) and cease to be victims of our unconscious actions.

Ayurveda was suppressed during the British rule of India for about 150 years. It survived in the remote rural countryside, where there was no other form of medical care. It is now blossoming, thanks in part, to the West's interest in natural, and holistic healing systems in which the whole person is considered, in the context of their environment, and their phase of life. Ayurveda also empowers the individual to take control of their health, through therapies and lifestyle practices like yoga and meditation that anyone can practice.

Ayurveda is mutable and has taken root in many different cultures over the years. It forms the basis of Tibetan medicine, and may have influenced Chinese medicine and the medicine of ancient Greece. It evolves with the times, such as incorporating surgical techniques. But the core of understanding your own body type and working towards harmony in your life has not changed.

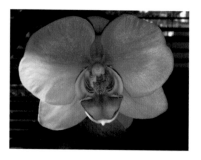

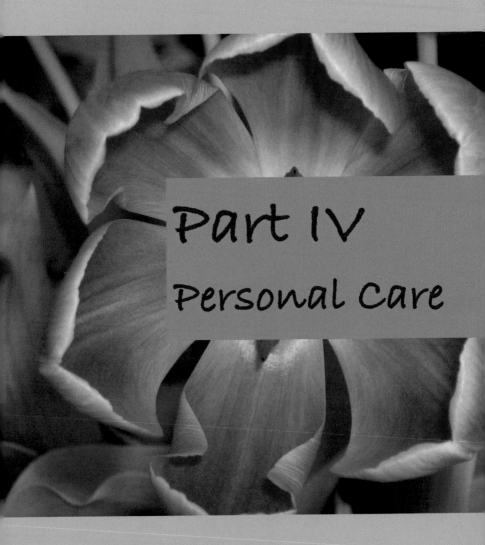

Part IV
Personal Care

Ergonomics

How do you use your body in the workplace?

Strategies for computer work

Take frequent breaks to move around

Change your chair positions and your mouse hand

Lean back when you are thinking or are on the phone

NEVER TYPE WITH THE PHONE CRADLED ON YOUR SHOULDER.

Invest in a headset— it's worth it

Look at a picture that has some depth,to change your focus

Have your hips higher than your knees

Avoid glare on the screen

Sitting still is not doing nothing. Small postural muscles are working hard to hold you in place, and they get very fatigued over time.

Executives used to have secretaries who took their dictation and even the secretaries had typewriters that had a built-in rest at the end of each line. But now everyone responds to their own email, many people spend 6 hours a day or more looking at computer screens and typing and using the mouse in one position all day long.

The areas that suffer the most are the neck, due to eyestrain, and the wrists and forearms and shoulders, due to the repetitive and static nature of typing. And laptops are the worst, since they make you conform your body to the machine. At least with a desktop you can adjust the height of the keyboard.

Simple exercises to do when you are taking your frequent 5 minute breaks (at least once an hour):

Exaggerated shoulder shrug
Lift your shoulders to your ears and let them drop slowly with a big exhalation (say "ha") 3—4 times. Lift and rotate your shoulders from front to back.

Flap your wings
Put your hands on your chest, lift and drop your elbows and see if you can get them to touch behind your back.

Pat yourself on the back
For a job well done!
Holding your upper right arm in your left hand, bring your right arm across your chest and pat your left shoulder. Then place your fingertips on the muscle on top of your shoulder and squeeze. Switch arms.

Eye cupping
Rub your palms together vigorously until you feel the heat build up between them. Then close your eyes and cup them with your warm palms for 20 seconds.

The most crucial aspect affecting arm and shoulder pain is the height of your keyboard.

Ideally, your shoulders should be relaxed and down, elbows bent, wrists straight (not flexed or hyperextended).

Your feet should be flat on the floor, your knees bent, your hips slightly higher than your knees, your lower back supported by your chair. Ideally your chair should be easily adjustable, and offer different, comfortable positions, like leaning back. Change positions often.
Change is good.

Know when to stop working

Massage Therapy

Muscle Tension

When a muscle is partially contracted, only some of the muscle fibers contract. For example, when you lift your shoulders slightly to reach the keyboard, some of the muscle fibers contract,and some do not. When you try to relax those muscles, some of the fibers stay contracted. By applying pressure, and bringing awareness, massage therapy can get those stubborn muscles to let go and relax completely.

Touch is essential for health. Infants die without it. Massage therapy can provide safe, skillful touch in this high tech world.

A good massage is like a guided tour through your body. From the delicacy of your little finger, to the depths of your trapezius, a skilled massage therapist will take you places you've never been. Your body becomes a like symphony for two. Massage therapy can release deeply held tension in your back and shoulders, increase circulation in your legs and feet, and reduce your level of anxiety and stress. When your body feels good, you feel better about life. It's a mini-vacation in an hour's time.

During the course of a massage, your breathing will naturally slow and deepen. The parasympathetic branch of your nervous system will take over, encouraging digestion and cellular repair. You will feel rejuvenated and rested with a sense of peace in body and mind. Massage therapy can be the perfect antidote to the stresses of modern life.

Benefits of massage therapy

★ increase relaxation
★ decrease stress
★ improve circulation
★ improve lymph flow
★ decrease anxiety
★ reduce muscle tension
★ improve mood
★ increase flexibility

Massage therapy is a great boost to the immune system. It's the only time that your lymph (the fluid surrounding cells) circulates without you moving and creating more waste products like lactic acid. Lymph fluid is moved along to lymph nodes where it is filtered.

There are almost as many kinds of massage as there are massage therapists. Try different people to see whom you like. You can find qualified therapists through The American Massage Therapy Association or The National Certification Board for Therapeutic Massage and Bodywork.

To find a massage therapist in your area: www.amatmassage.org or www.ncbtmb.org or www.massage.com

Types of Massage

Swedish massage: pleasant, relaxing stroking and kneading of muscles; directing blood flow back to the heart

Deep tissue massage: more pressure to reach the deeper layers of muscles and connective tissue

Acupressure: finger pressure used on acupuncture points to stimulate the flow of chi energy

Shiatsu: a rhythmic form of acupressure

Craniosacral: very light fingertip touch on the head and sacrum, very relaxing

Myofacial release: a deep stretching of the facia, the connective tissue that surrounds the muscles, good for resolving trauma

Bodywork

Bodywork generally refers to manual manipulation that is deeper than massage, and aims to alter your structural alignment

Rolfing

Ida Rolf and Moishe Feldenkrais were friends at Esalen Institute at Big Sur in the early 1970s. Ida Rolf called her work "Structural Integration". She was interested in the fascia, the connective tissue that covers all of the muscles.

Rolfing is done in a series of ten sessions to improve posture and alignment and one's relationship to gravity. It is a very deep, slow form of bodywork.

http://www.rolf.org/

Feldenkrais

Moishe Feldenkrais was born in Russia, traveled extensively, trained in Judo and mechanical engineering. He suffered a knee injury playing soccer and developed his method as rehabilitation.

"Awareness Through Movement," is a class taught to groups to increase neuromotor and sensory awareness. Using small movements and verbal cues, students are led through a series of movements and ways of thinking that highlight our habitual ways of moving and introduce new possibilities.

"Functional Integration" is taught one-on-one using gentle touch and movements to increase the range of the students movements. Feldenkrais is beneficial for everyone, but especially good for injuries where there is restriction in range of motion, or strain from repetitive movements.

http://www.feldenkrais.com/

Hanna Somatics

Thomas Hanna, the creator of "Somatics" died tragically in a car accident. When the police found his body, they thought he was a man in his forties, but he was actually 62 years old when he died. He left us an excellent book, <u>Somatics</u>, that explains his life's work.

He studied with Feldenkrais and brought him to the United States for the first time. Hanna developed the work even further and named it "Hanna Somatic Education"

We get stuck in patterns of movement, which he named the "green light reflex" and the "red light reflex." Certain postural muscles shorten over time with this habitual use, resulting in the stooped forward posture of old age. He claims that if we do some of his simple exercises every day we can maintain our flexibility and youthful posture. www.hannasomatics.com

a sample exercise:
"Lying on your back, arch and flatten your lower back, inhaling while going up and exhaling while going down. Repeat five times over thirty seconds." Move slowly like a cat."

Hanna, Thomas. <u>Somatics</u>

Home remedies

Strains and Sprains

Strains are an injury to the tendons, the connective tissue that connects the **muscles to the bones.**

Sprains injure the ligaments, the connective tissue that **connects bones to bones.**

If it hurts when you use your muscles, but not when you move the area passively, (like when someone moves it for you) then it's a strain.

If it hurts when you move an area passively (without using your muscles) chances are it's a sprain.

You will want to start moving the area as soon as you can without pain, but not bearing weight. Moving the injured body part, but not stressing it, will help prevent excessive scar tissue and adhesions (when scar tissue adheres to bones). It will also increase blood circulation and avoid atrophy (weakening of the muscle).

Traditional treatment
RICE=
rest
ice
compression
elevation
For severe injuries
New treatment
MICE=
movement,
ice
compression
elevation
is now recommended for most soft tissue injuries

Ice is a very effective treatment, used as soon as possible after the injury. It promotes a deeper blood circulation, driving the blood away from the surface of the body and slowing the accumulation of inflammatory products (inflammation slows down blood flow) and it also relieves pain, allowing you to move the area gently.

Hendrickson, Thomas. <u>Massage for Orthopedic Conditions.</u>

Common Strains

Ankles are often sprained by stumbling and turning the foot inward. Apply ice right away. After the injury has healed, a good exercise for a sprained ankle is to write the alphabet in the air with your toes. You want to strengthen the area during the remodeling phase of injury (about 4 weeks after the initial injury, lasting up to a year thereafter).

Another area that is often strained and sprained from a fall is the **wrist**. You want to initially immobilize it to commence healing, but you want to start making small movements in one direction only and then back to center, as soon as pain allows. Light massage can help relieve the swelling.

Back strain occurs by lifting too much weight, or lifting in an awkward position. Rest, ice and ibuprofen (about 600 mg every 4-6 hours for 72 hours) can be effective for pain relief. Find a position of comfort: either lying flat on the floor on a mat; or lying on your stomach in a slight cobra position (head raised, slightly elbows bent under shoulders, forearms flat on the floor) can be helpful; lying on one side, one knee up supported by a pillow; or both knees up, fetal position. Sleeping on the floor with a thick mat can give you a feeling of support, that can help back spasms. After the injury has healed, strengthening the abdominal muscles can help support your back.

Neck strain can be helped by placing a rolled up towel inside your pillowcase while you sleep. Start with a small hand towel or dish towel, and experiment to what's most comfortable for you.

When to use ice

❊ At the start of an injury, the first 24-48 hours, the sooner the better. Promotes deeper circulation, driving the blood away from the surface of the skin.

❊ Provides pain relief, making the area numb. You can move the injured area gently, which helps the area heal, and the scar tissue to properly form.

❊ Ice massage can be done with ice in a styrofoam cup. Keep the ice moving over your skin, for about 20 minutes/ session.
A towel can be dipped in ice water and replaced as it warms.

Ice therapy is not recommended if you have rheumatoid arthritis, diabetes, or allergy to cold. Be careful moving when you are numb from the ice, that you do not injure yourself further!

When to use heat

❋ After the acute stage of an injury has passed, about 48 hours.

❋ For relaxing tense muscles.

❋ For menstrual cramps.

❋ For stress reduction, for whole body relaxation.

Hot baths with epson salts are helpful for muscle fatigue.

Moist heat packs penetrate better than dry electric heating pads.

Herbal heat packs that you can heat in the microwave are convenient.

Hot + cold therapy
1 minute of cold + 4 minutes of heat =5 minutes. Repeat 4 times for a 20 minute treatment. Then rest, to let circulation normalize.

Colds & Flu

Colds start as a little tickle in the back of your throat. Then your throat is sore, and that little tickle feeling moves up into your sinuses, or down into your chest. It takes a little while to really get going, a day or two. Treat it aggressively at the beginning and you may be able to catch it before it starts.

Influenza or "the flu" is a stronger virus than a cold virus. It hits you all at once. You have no choice but to rest. Your body feels achy all over. You don't feel like eating anything. The hot lemon and honey toddy can be soothing.

You have to marvel at our bodies ability to recognize this invader and to to fight it off. Modern medicine doesn't have anything as sophisticated as our immune system.

A fever is a good thing; it's your body's way of fighting the infection. A fever below 104° needs no medication. Above 105°, call the doctor. A cool washcloth can be soothing. Let your body fight the infection, drink water to stay hydrated.

Humor can be helpful. Think positive thoughts. Rest and let your body heal.

http://www.mayoclinic.com/health/fever

Home remedies for colds

Gargle with warm salt water, morning and evening. About a teaspoon of salt in half a cup of warm water can really help you get over a cold. It soothes a sore throat and it kills bacteria (remember salt was used as a preservative.)

Zinc lozenges with vitamin C. The zinc coats your throat and it makes it more difficult for the virus to take hold. Vitamin C strengthens cell membranes.

Hot lemon and honey toddy. Squeeze half a lemon and one heaping teaspoon of honey into two cups of hot water. You can drink this throughout the duration of your cold. You can add a tablespoon of brandy at night to help you sleep. Skip the brandy if you are taking other medications that make you drowsy.

My father used to say, "Whiskey when you're well makes you sick, whiskey when you're sick makes you well." Don't add it if you have a problem with alcohol.

Fresh garlic is a good natural antibiotic. An easy way to take it is to chop up one clove and spread it on buttered toast . You can top it with honey if you like. Or in scrambled eggs adding the fresh garlic at the last moment of cooking. Raw garlic is the most therapeutic, as heat destroys some of its potency. If your throat is really sore, try sucking on a whole peeled clove, chewing little bits at a time. Best when you don't have social engagements planned!

Ginger tea. Grate fresh ginger (1- inch piece) into 2 cups of water, simmer for 20 minutes. If your nose is stuffed, put a towel over your head, lean over the pot after it has simmered and breathe in the steam. After it's cooled down, add honey and drink the tea.

Rest as much as you can. Give your body a chance to recognize the virus and produce antibodies to it. Remember, your body fights infection better when it's not under stress.

Coughs

There are wet productive coughs (where phlegm comes up) and dry hacking irritating coughs where nothing comes up. Usually the wet cough is first and this is the kind of cough you want to encourage. It's your body's way of getting the mucus up and out of your lungs. Steaming with the ginger tea (see above) or steaming with just plain water can be helpful. Just relax and breathe deeply, let the heat relax your bronchioles.

The other kind of cough, dry and hacking after the initial illness has passed, doesn't do much good. There are cough suppressants out there, but I find caffeine can be helpful. Black tea with lots of honey can be a good bronchial dilator, or sucking on cough drops can help. Warm brandy can be helpful at night. In a pinch, homemade cough syrup can be made using one teaspoon of honey and a tablespoon of brandy. This is also a good time to get extra rest, so your body can finish its clean-up job.

There is a saying that a cold lasts seven days and if you go to the doctor, it lasts a week. It's a process that your body has to go through, but you can make it easier by resting and letting your body concentrate on getting well.

Homemade cough syrup
1 tsp. honey
1 Tbl. brandy

Part V
Mind/Body

Healthy habits can be challenged by short-term pleasure seeking drives. One fix is to substitute healthy alternatives. Dark chocolate has more health-giving properties than milk chocolate. You can train yourself to like dark chocolate and choose it over milk chocolate.

You can reward yourself with an extra lap in the pool, or a five-minute longer walk. Change your mental construct of exercise as a chore, and instead see it as a reward.

Power down

Sometimes you have to turn the computer off, give it a break, and then it works better. The same is true with us. We need breaks from our routine to be renewed. Sometimes it's taking a different route to work, or taking a vacation, or just taking a walk in nature to renew our spirits. We need to make sure we have mini breaks throughout the day, even if it's just a two minute break to close our eyes and breathe.

When you come home from work, design a ritual where you have ten or fifteen minutes of transition time: Lie on your yoga mat for a few minutes and relax. If you have young children or animals, they'll think it's the greatest thing. Cats, especially, will think that you've come to your senses.

Unplug

Sometimes we have to unplug. We are constantly bombarded with news we can't use. But sometimes we need to turn off the TV and the computer, and have a "news fast." Maybe we'll get some new insight on how to help the state of the world.

Worry date

Spend a fixed amount of time planning for your week, say 15 minutes on Sunday evening. Worry about everything you need to worry about, write it down, if you must, and then stop worrying.

Dr. Marty Rossman, a guided imagery expert, says worrying is, "unguided imagery." Instead, visualize what you want to see happening. Use as much detail as possible.

When you have stressful, worried thoughts, your body is responding to those, too. When you spend a lot of time getting prepared, getting geared up, your body prepares too, by activating the stress hormone cascade (CRH-ACTH-cortisol) and getting you ready for fight-or-flight. If you respond to everyday life, as if it is an emergency, you will wear yourself down.

Experience how your body responds to your thoughts (after you read this, close your eyes and try it for yourself)

In your mind's eye, imagine seeing a big juicy yellow lemon. Now imagine taking a knife and cutting the lemon in half. Smell the tangy, fresh lemon scent. Now imagine bringing half of that lemon up to your mouth and tasting it. What is happening right now in your mouth? Are you starting to salivate?

Your body responds to your mind.

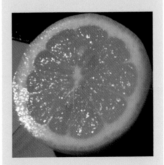

Ways to be happy

Laughter Yoga

Laughing any time for any reason is good for your system

★Increases oxygen intake

★Decreases stress hormones

★Improves cardiovascular function

★Improves mood

There are laughter clubs forming all over the world

Flow: when you are really engrossed in something, engaged, but not overwhelmed. When your sense of time goes quickly. It is fantastic if your work feels like this. It's good if you can find a hobby that makes you feel this way.

Creativity: an important part of a full life. Find some means of self-expression. Writing, drawing, playing music, cooking, sewing, photography, carpentry. Painting with watercolors can be fun; doodling in color. Let the right side of your brain, the side that handles images, not words, be in charge once in a while.

Gratitude: keep a gratitude journal. Write down things that you are grateful for each day. Remind yourself of good times in your life. Recreate them in your mind. Let yourself bask in the beach of your mind.

http://www.laughteryoga.org/   Mihály Csíkszentmihályi, Flow

Begin watching your thoughts, so you can see what's going on.
See what kinds of signals you are sending to your body.
Monitor the content and the emotional tone of your thoughts.

Just by paying attention and watching your thoughts go by,
they will change.

You'll be able to spot obsessive or reoccurring negative
thoughts by labeling them:"There's a thought about the future,"
or "That's a to-do list," or "That's something from the past."

Bring your attention to the present moment by focusing on
your breath.

You can challenge negative thoughts by replacing them with
sayings like "One day at a time," or "This too shall pass."

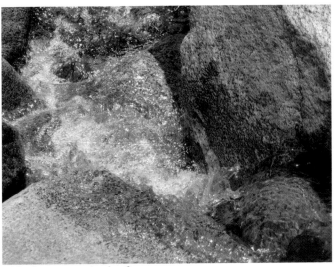

Life is a rough draft

You don't have to be perfect

They call it meditation "practice"

Ingredients for a happy life

★ good health
★ friends
★ family
★ community
★ safety
★ meaningful work
★ enough money
★ feeling valued
★ giving to others
★ connection to Self, Source, God, Spirit, whatever you want to call it
★ hope for the future

You can choose to be happy— find what brings *you* joy

How you frame it for yourself, is the way things are for you.

Be happy
Be healthy

Pleasure and Happiness

Pleasure is fleeting, a sensation that cannot last. It is a delight in something outside of ourselves, a momentary diversion. The pleasure centers of the brain light up, flare for a moment, and then we want more: drugs, sugar, excitement, whatever.

But happiness is different. It comes from inside of ourselves. Different areas of the brain light up (the left frontal cortex) where feelings of well-being arise. When we have a feeling of inner peace, then we are not so bound up with our circumstances.

Studies have shown that lottery winners, after the initial euphoria wears off, are as about as happy as they were before they won the money. Conversely, people who become disabled after an accident, after a period of adjustment, are just a little less happy than they were before the injury. We seem to have a "set-point" for happiness, that circumstances do not change.

But can we "learn" how to be happy? Happy people are healthier. And live longer. And have a better time.

Seligman, Martin. Authentic Happiness

Monk's Brains

Experienced meditators, Tibetan monks, were brought into the laboratory and their brain waves were measured while they meditated. Their left prefrontal cortex showed significant activity, an area associated with happiness, and positive thoughts and feelings. The right pre-frontal cortex, associated with negative emotions and anxiety, was less activated.

They also produced deep gamma waves, deeper than anyone had ever seen, indicating higher consciousness. When they did "loving kindness" meditation the motor skills part of their brain fired up, as if they couldn't wait to get started helping others.

Neuroplasticity
Your brain changes in response to experience and thoughts

Mental training
You can train your brain, by paying attention to your thoughts and feelings

Practice
feeling compassion and gratitude

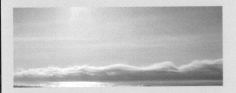

Just
 be
present

Begley, Sharon. "Scans of Monks' Brains Show Meditation Alters Structure, Functioning" <u>Wall Street Journal</u> 5November2004

Mindfulness is being aware

of the present

of what is going on in your mind

Being present in your body
paying attention to what is

Examining the content of your
thoughts, but not getting caught
up in them

Developing the witness that
sees the thoughts

Releasing judgement
just being present with what is

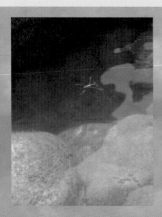

Really being present for your life
Fully engaged in the moment

Awake   131

Guided visualization
Sit in a comfortable place or lie down

Close your eyes and imagine sitting in a movie theatre. In your mind's eye imagine there is a blank screen and on that screen imagine seeing a red square. See the top and bottom and sides of that red square. See it change into a cube and examine all the sides of the cube.

Now let that cube dissolve and in its place see a triangle, a green triangle, and see all three sides of the green triangle. Let the triangle dissolve and in its place see an orange circle— rising like the sun from the bottom of the screen. And now it rises like the sun and you can feel the heat from this sun. Now you can imagine yourself walking along a path, you can feel the gravel crunching beneath your feet, you can hear birds singing in the distance, you can sense the warm sun on your face and feel a gentle breeze on your cheek.

Now this path takes you along a riverbank, and you walk along hearing the gentle murmur of the water. You see a bench and you sit down to rest. In the distance you see familiar figures coming towards you, dear friends, and you are glad to see them. They have something they want to tell you, some wisdom to impart. You listen, stay as long as is comfortable, and then you see the sun is starting to set and it's time to bring yourself back. Count up slowly from 1 to 5 and when you reach the number 5 you are back in your chair.

reverie, like doodling, is hearing from the right side of the brain... images, other kinds of wisdom. Listen

Body scan

Before meditation:
   Bring your attention to your feet. See how your feet are feeling today. Bring your attention to your calves, your thighs, hips. Feel where your bottom is contacting the cushion or the chair. Bring your awareness to your lower back, mid back, upper back, shoulders. Feel any tension in your shoulders? Raise them slightly and let them drop, and let the tension melt away with the next out breath. Bring your awareness to your neck. Let your neck relax. Bring your awareness to your scalp, your eyelids. Let all your tension go.

Meditation

   Sit comfortably. Let your belly be soft. Breathe easily. Bring your attention to your breath. Watch your breath. Bring your awareness to the tip of your nose. Notice the breath coming in. Notice the breath going out. Let any thoughts you have drift by like clouds. Bring your attention back to your breath. At first it can be helpful to have a timer, so you don't have to be concerned about the time. Start with ten minutes. When your mind wanders, bring your attention back to your breath.

Balance

Everyone needs balance in their lives. Balance of work, family, and personal time. Balance of exercise and rest. Balance of healthy eating and occasional indulgence.

Everyone has their own particular constitution. We all need different amounts of sleep, and different foods to nourish us at different times of the day. A little caffeine may be appropriate early in the day, not so good past 4 o'clock. Some people do better having a little meat in their diet (grass-fed beef would be best, due to higher omega-3 content).

Eat to suit the season, more raw vegetables and fresh fruit in warmer weather, more soups and stews, and cooked foods in the colder months.
"Flexitarian" (flexible) is an optimal approach to food. After all, we are omnivores, we have the teeth to eat meat and grains.

Find the kind of exercise that's right for you, that you enjoy, that you look forward to.

Take the time to be present in your life. Breathe deeply.

Find the time each day to:
stretch
relax
breathe
smile
laugh

Positive emotions reduce stress

Find community and nourish your connection with other people

Take refuge in the moment

Explaining Health Recommendations

✓ Breathe—let your belly be soft and exhale completely and then breathe in deeply
✓ Relax—give yourself permission
✓ Sleep—make it a priority
✓ Fish oil—be sure to get adequate omega-3
✓ Green tea—drink up to 5 cups a day for the protective antioxidants
✓ Use olive oil in place of butter
✓ Yoga mat—everyone should own a yoga mat and spend some time each day, moving and stretching on the floor
✓ Walk!—brisk walking can improve cardiovascular health
✓ Swimming is wonderful exercise
✓ Epsom salt baths—for muscular aches and pains
✓ Microwave heat packs—for relaxation and muscular pain
✓ Foam rollers can help relieve muscular tension
✓ Schedule regular massage therapy
✓ Be open to change—life is like surfing, sometimes you lose your balance, and you have to get up again
✓ Be of service—find ways to give to others
✓ Find your community and actively participate

References

Santrock, John W.Life Span Development ,McGraw Hill © 2006

National Center for Health Statistics, www.cdc.gov/nchs/faststas/lifexpec.htm 7/16/05

Weil, Andrew, MD.Healthy Aging a Lifelong Guide to Your Physical and Spiritual Well-Being Knopf © 2005

Wilcox, Bradley.The Okinawa Program: how the worlds longest -lived people achieve everlasting health-and how you can too.Three River Press .© 2001

Anderson, Norman B., Ph.D. Emotional Longevity What Really Determines How Long You Live-.Viking-Penguin Group. © 2003

Sapolsky, Robert M.Why Zebras Don't Get Ulcers An Updated Guide to Stress, Stress-Related Diseases and Coping -W.H. Freeman © 2000

Napastek, Bellaruth. Staying Well with Guided Imagery"

Seligman Martin E. P., Ph.d. Learned Optimism How to Change your life and your mind and Authentic Happiness Simon & Shuster ©. 2002

Piscatella, Joseph.Take A Load Off Your Heart 109 things You Can Actually Do to Prevent, Halt and Reverse heart Disease, Workman Publishing © 2003

Thondup, Tulku.The Healing Power of Mind, Simple Meditation Exercises for Health, Well-Being and Enlightenment by, Shambala Publications © 1996

Bailey, Covert.The New Fit or Fat, Houghton Mifflin © 1991

Benjamin, Ben, Ph.D. Listen to Your Pain, The active person's Guide to Understanding, Identifying, and Treating Pain and Injury. Penguin Books © 1984

Hendrickson, Thomas DC. Massage for Orthopedic Conditions Institute of Orthopedic Massage. Lippincott, Williams and Wilkens © 2003

Environmental Working Group http://www.ewg.org/

Trivieri, Larry, Jr.The American Holistic Medical Association's Guide to Holistic Health. John Wiley &Sons © 2001

Beinfield &Korngold, A.Ac. Between Heaven and Earth-AGuide to Chinese Medicine, Ballentine Books, 1991

Lad, Vasant, M.A.Sc.Textbook of Ayurveda Fundamental Principles, Ayurvedic Press, 2002

Moyers, Bill. Healing and the Mind, Doubleday, 1993

CPSIA information can be obtained
at www.ICGtesting.com
Printed in the USA
LVIC04n1207180414
382298LV00001B/1